PROSTATE CANCER IN QUESTIONS

Treatment

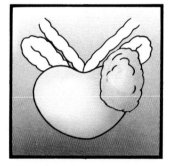

S. KHOURY · C. CHATELAIN · G. MURPHY · L. DENIS
P. MECHALI

SCI

Preface

This book is designed to help urologists and other specialists working in the field of prostate cancer in their **everyday practice**.

The treatment of prostatic cancer is certainly the most controversial subject in the field of urology and it is very difficult to write a didactic and practical guide on this subject.

Discussing the treatment modalities of prostatic cancer remains a rather easy and pleasant academic exercise as long as we don't have to act. Action is "all or nothing " and requires a definite stand.

We are thus aware that **any recommendation** in relation to a given situation **is inevitably schematic** and cannot be applied universally. On the other hand, a more complete view may tend to confuse the message and make it unusable in clinical practice .

For this reason, for the more controversial subjects, in addition to the principal "schematic" article, we have presented the **opinions of various authors** recognised for their work in this field, in order to help the reader to reach a more precise opinion and to manage his patients acccording to the most up-to-date knowledge.

To achieve a more homogeneous presentation, we have used, whenever possible, the "**New TNM**" classification, although the **Whitmore classification** has been used in a few articles . A **comparative table** of the TNM and Whitmore classifications is presented on page 10.

We would like to thank all those who have contributed to this book and we are confident that it will achieve its objective .

It is said that " one book more is one forest less". Although we try to use recycled paper whenever possible we hope that the benefit to public health of this book more than offsets the harm of cutting down a few trees !

The Scientific Committee

AUTHORS

AUSTENFELD M.S.
Division of Urology
University of Kansas Medical Center
Kansas City
USA

BAGSHAW M.A.
Department of Radiation Oncology
Stanford University - School of Medicine
Stanford
USA

BAZINET M.
Urology Department
The Sloan Kettering Memorial Hospital
New York
USA

BEISLAND H.O.
Department of Urology
Aker Hospital
Oslo
NORWAY

BORLAND R.N.
The James Buchanan Urological Institute
The Johns Hopkins Medical Institutions
Baltimore
USA

BRENDLER C.B.
James Buchanan Brady Urology Institute
The Johns Hopkins Medical Institutions
Baltimore
USA

BRESSEL M.
Allgemeines Krankenhaus Harburg
Urologische Abteilung
Hamburg
GERMANY

CARLTON C.E.
Department of Urology
Baylor College of Medicine
Houston
USA

CATALONA W.J.
Division of Urologic Surgery
Washington University Medical Center
Saint Louis
USA

CHATELAIN C.
Clinique Urologique
Hôpital de la Pitié
Paris
FRANCE

DENIS L.
President of the International
Prostate Health Council
Department of Urology - AZ Middelheim
Anvers, BELGIUM

FLYNN D.F.
Department of Radiation Medicine
Massachussetts General Hospital Cancer
Boston
USA

FRAZIER H.A.
Division of Urology
Duke University Medical Center
Durham
USA

GRIFFITHS K.
Department of Urology
St. Woolos and Royal Gwent Hospitals
Newport, Gwent
UK

HORWICH A.
Department of Radiotherapy & Oncology
The Royal Marsden Hospital
Sutton, Surrey
USA

HUDSON P.B.
Department of Urology
University of South Florida
Florida
USA

KAPLAN I.D.
Department of Radiation & Oncology
Stanford University School of Medicine
Saint Louis
USA

KAVOUSSI L.
Division of Urologic Surgery
Washington University School of Medicine
Saint Louis
USA

KHOURY S.
Urology Department
Hôpital de la Pitié
Paris
FRANCE

LANGE P.
Department of Urology
University of Washington Medical Center
Seattle
USA

LINK P.
Division of Urology
Stanford University Medical School
Stanford
USA

LYNCH J.H.
Division of Urology
Georgetown University
Washington
USA

MECHALI P.
Urology Department
Hôpital Louise Michel
Evry
FRANCE

MIDDLETON R.G.
Division of Urology - Dep. of Surgery
Uni. of Utah Cent. for the Health Sciences
Salt Lake City
USA

MONTIE J.E.
Department of Urology
Cleveland Clinic Florida
Florida
USA

MORTON R.
The James Buchanan Brady Urol. Institute
The Johns Hopkins Medical Institutions
Baltimore
USA

MURPHY G.
Vice Président
American Cancer Society
Atlanta
USA

PARA k.
Division of Urology
St Louis University School of Medecine
Saint Louis
USA

PAULSON D.F.
Division of Urology
Duke University Medical Center
Durham
USA

PETROS J.A.
Division of Urologic Surgery
Washington University School of Medecine
Saint Louis
USA

PICHARD LEANDRI E.
Unité de Diagnostic et Trait. de la douleur
Institut Gustave Roussy
Villejuif
FRANCE

QUINLAN D.
Saint Vincent's Hospital

Dublin
IRELAND

RIGONDET G.
Polyclinique St. François

Montluçon
FRANCE

ROBERT M.
Department of Urology

Egertsville
USA

ROSSIGNOL G.
Service Urologie
Saint Jean Languedoc-Cerou
Toulouse
FRANCE

RUSSELL K.J.
Departments of Radiation & Oncology
University of Washington
Seattle
USA

SCHELLHAMMER P.F.
Department of Urology
Eastern Virginia Medical School
Norfolk
USA

SHIPLEY W.U.
Department of Radiation Medicine
Massachussetts General Hosp. Cancer Cent.
Boston
USA

SMITH J.A.
Division of Urology
University of Utah
Salt Lake City
USA

SMITH P.H.
Department of Urology
Saint. James University Hospital
Leeds
UK

SOLE BALCELLS F.
Fundacion Puigvert

Barcelona
SPAIN

STUDER U.E.
Inselspital
Urologishe Universitätsklinik
Bern
Switzerland

VICENTE J.
Fundation Puigvert

Barcelona
SPAIN

VOGES G.E.
Division of Urology
Stanford University School of Medicine
Stanford
USA

WHITMORE W.F.
Urologic Service
Sloan Kettering Cancer Center
New York
USA

ZINCKE H.
Department of Urology and Surgery
Mayo Clinic
Rochester
USA

CONTENTS

METHODS

I. Radical Surgery

INDICATIONS

CLASSIFICATION

Table 1. Classification of prostatic cancer

Whitmore 1956[2]
(with modifications)
Stage   TNM 1992[4]

Whitmore stage	TNM
	T0 No evidence of primary tumour
A Not palpable on rectal exam	**T1** Clinically inapparent tumour, not palpable and not visible by imaging
A1 Focal cancer (<3 chips)	**T1a** Tumour an incidental histological finding in ≤5% of tissue resected
A2 Diffuse (>3 chips)	**T1b** Tumour an incidental histological finding in >5% of tissue resected
	T1c Tumour identified by needle biopsy (e.g. because of elevated serum PSA)
B B1 Unilobar, <2 cm	**T2** Tumour confined within the prostate ●
	T2a Tumour involves half of a lobe or less
B2 Unilobar, >2 cm	**T2b** Tumour involves more than half a lobe but not both lobes
B3 All other, intracapsular	**T2c** Tumour involves both lobes
C Extending through capsule	**T3** Tumour extends through the prostatic capsule ▲
C1 Sulcus or sulci not free	
C2 >Base of seminal vesicles ± sulci	**T3a** Unilateral extracapsular extension
	T3b Bilateral extracapsular extension
	T3c Tumour invades seminal vesicle(s)
C3 >Base of seminal vesicles ± other adjacent organs	**T4** Tumour fixed or invades adjacent structures other than seminal vesicles
	T4a Tumour invades bladder neck and/or external sphincter and/or rectum
	T4b Tumour invades levator muscles and/or is fixed to pelvic wall
D Any local extension	
D1 Lymph node involvement	
D2 Other metastases	

● Tumour found in one or both lobes by needle biopsy, but not palpable or visible by imaging, is classified as T1c
▲ Invasion into the prostatic apex or into (but not beyond) the prostatic capsule is not classified as T3 but as T2

Schröder FH, Hermanek P, Denis L, Fair WR, Gospodarowicz, Pavone-Macaluso M. The TNM classification of prostate carcinoma. *Prostate* 1992; Suppl 4:129–38

Prostate : Clinical Classification

					N+	%PAP	%PSA
Incidental	A1	T1a	Incidental histologic findings in 5% or less of tissue resected		2		
	A2	T1b	Incidental histologic findings in more than 5% of tissue resected			12	20
		T1c	Tumor identified by needle biopsy (e.g., because of elevated PSA)		23		
Organ Confined	B1	T2a	Tumor involves half of a lobe or less		18		
	B2	T2b	Tumor involves more than half a lobe but not both lobes			30	40
	B3	T1c	Tumor involves both lobes		35		
Locally Invasive	C1	T3a	Unilateral extracapsular extension	T4 tumor is fixed or invades adjacent structures other than seminal vesicles	50		
		T3b	Bilateral extracapsular extension			45	70
	C2	T3c	Tumor invades seminal vesicle (s)	T4	80		
Dissemi-nated	D1	N+			100		
						90	92
	D2	M+			—		
	D3	Resistant to hormone therapy					

11

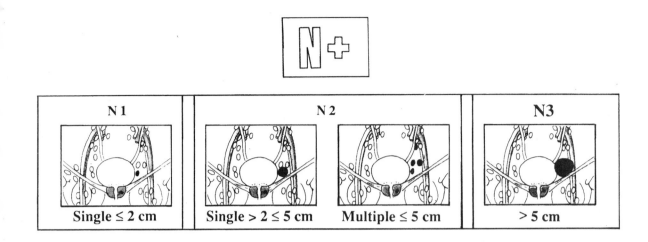

CLASSIFICATION

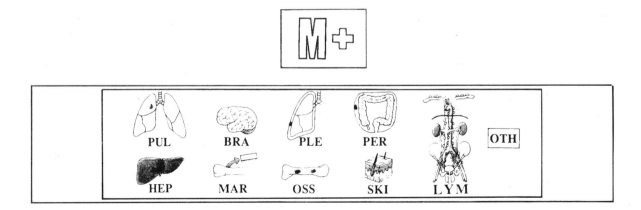

I

METHODS

.

SURGERY

Surgical Technique of Retropubic Radical Prostatectomy

G. Rossignol
Toulouse, France

I . PATIENT PREPARATION

1. Preparation prior to the operation

Surgery is performed an average of 6 to 8 weeks after prostatic needle biopsy, but it is perfectly possible to operate during the week after the prostatic biopsy, provided there is no haematoma or prostatitis.

Transfusions are rarely necessary with meticulous intraoperative haemostasis, but if the patient refuses heterologous transfusion, autologous transfusion can be proposed and 3 units of blood can be collected during the month preceding the operation, or normovolemic hemodilution can be performed on the day before the operation.

The patient is prepared 48 hours before the operation by a low residue diet, enema in the evening before the operation and antibiotics consisting of an anti-anaerobic antibiotic for 48 hours before the operation and a 3rd generation cephalosporin on call to the operating room.

2. Operative preparation

Special instruments : the operation is facilitated by using instruments adapted to prostatectomy : Balfour's retractor with a large midline valve, long instruments with curved scissors and an angled needle-holder.

Anaesthesia : spinal or peridural anaesthesia is often performed, but we do not believe that it alters the postoperative course in comparison with general anaesthesia, as the two most important points are the duration of the operation and the blood losses.

II . OPERATIVE TECHNIQUE

The operative technique has been previously described and has been modified by Walsh .

1. The patient is placed in the ***dorsal supine position*** and, during access to the urethra, the table is broken and tilted 20° in a Trendelenburg position. A suprapubic extraperitoneal midline incision is made. The vasa deferentes are sectioned and the spermatic pedicles are preserved.

2. *Pelvic lymph node dissection* is performed cautiously and is limited to the medial nodes of the external iliac chain, the obturator nodes and the nodes at the external and internal iliac bifurcation. Lymphostasis is ensured by non-absorbable clips and ligatures. All of the nodes removed are submitted to frozen section pathological examination.

3. *Radical prostatectomy is then performed* according to perfectly defined stages.

a. Incision of the endo-pelvic fascia (Figures 1 and 2)

b. Urethral part (Figures 3 to 7)

c. Dissection of the posterior surface of the prostate (Figures 8 and 9)

d. Vesical part (Figures 10, 11 and 12)

e. Vesicourethral anastomosis (Figure 13)

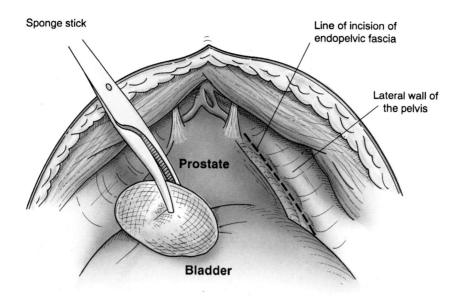

Figure 1 : Pelvic lymph node dissection has been performed. Radical prostatectomy starts with incision of the endopelvic fascia with a scalpel blade at the postero-inferior part of the fascia on the line of reflection against the pelvic wall.

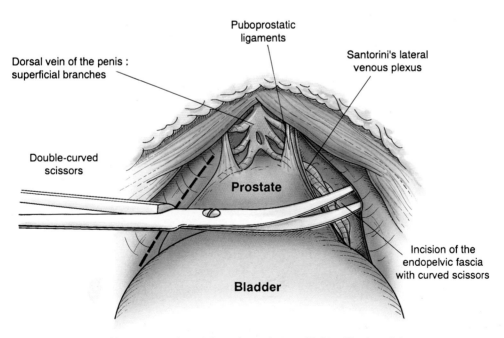

Figure 2 : Simple spreading of the scissors helps with identification of the proper plane of cleavage and allows the completion of the fascial incision up to the puboprostatic ligament anteriorly. At this stage the field must be bloodless ; it allows exploration of the lateral walls of the prostate and, anteriorly, assessment of the thickness of the puboprostatic ligaments and fascia covering the apex of the prostate, between the thumb and index finger.

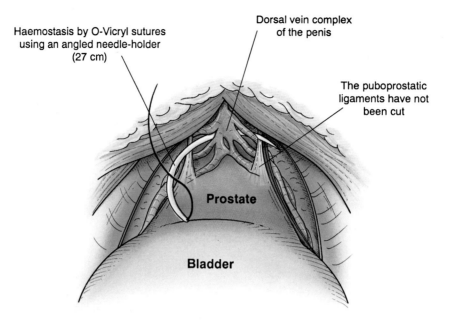

Figure 3 : The puboprostatic ligaments are only cut at their insertion onto the pubis when the incision can be made easily without dissection and with no risk of injury to the superficial dorsal vein. In general, haemostasis of the superficial dorsal vein is ensured by a Vicryl suture which includes the puboprostatic ligaments.

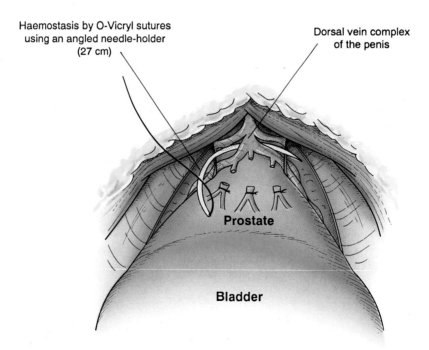

Figure 4 : 3 or 4 sutures allow the anterior surface of the urethra to be reached while avoiding any blood loss and preserving as much of anterior periurethral fascia as possible.

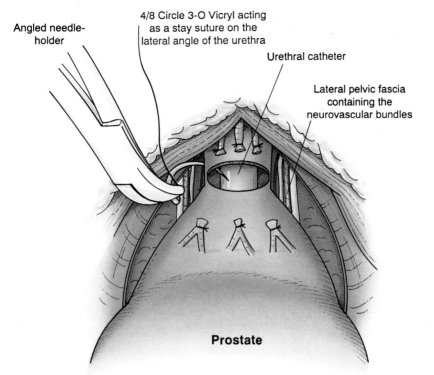

Angled needle-holder

4/8 Circle 3-O Vicryl acting as a stay suture on the lateral angle of the urethra

Urethral catheter

Lateral pelvic fascia containing the neurovascular bundles

Prostate

Figure 5 : The anterior surface of the urethra is sectioned at the level of the prostato-urethral junction and 2 3-O Vicryl sutures are passed over the urethra for identification and presentation of the urethra and are subsequently used for the vesicourethral anastomosis. During nerve-sparing procedures, great care must be taken to avoid injury to the lateral pelvic fascia containing the neurovascular bundles.

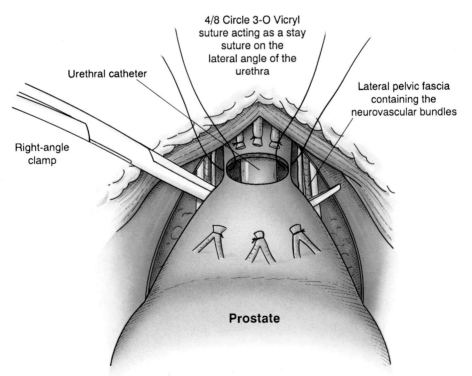

4/8 Circle 3-O Vicryl suture acting as a stay suture on the lateral angle of the urethra

Urethral catheter

Lateral pelvic fascia containing the neurovascular bundles

Right-angle clamp

Prostate

Figure 6 : Fine dissecting scissors open up a plane very close to the lateral wall of the urethra and separate the urethra from the lateral pelvic fascia. A right-angle clamp is inserted into this plane of dissection to free the urethra.

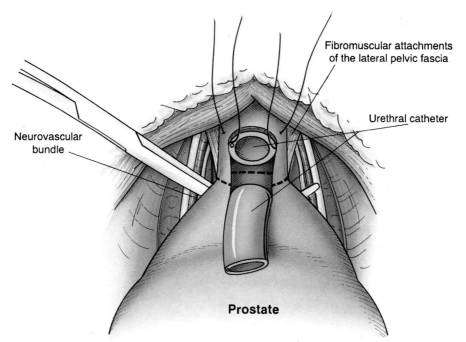

Figure 7 : Section of the posterior wall of the urethra controlled by a right-angle dissector in order to preserve as much urethral length as possible and to protect the neurovascular bundles, lying posteriorly.

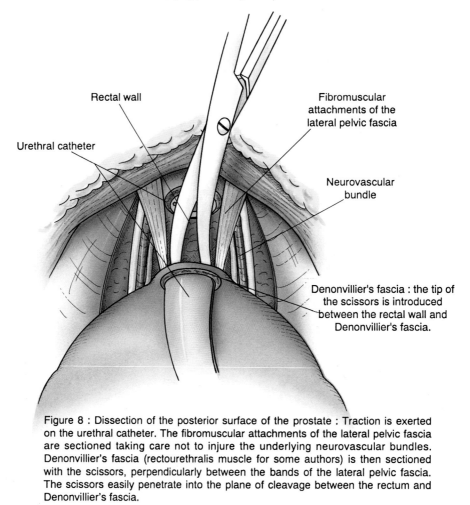

Figure 8 : Dissection of the posterior surface of the prostate : Traction is exerted on the urethral catheter. The fibromuscular attachments of the lateral pelvic fascia are sectioned taking care not to injure the underlying neurovascular bundles. Denonvillier's fascia (rectourethralis muscle for some authors) is then sectioned with the scissors, perpendicularly between the bands of the lateral pelvic fascia. The scissors easily penetrate into the plane of cleavage between the rectum and Denonvillier's fascia.

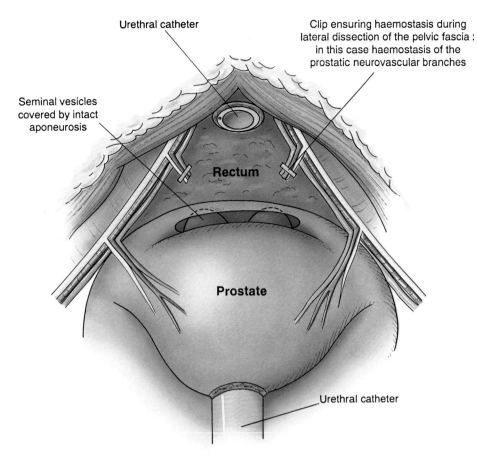

Urethral catheter

Clip ensuring haemostasis during lateral dissection of the pelvic fascia : in this case haemostasis of the prostatic neurovascular branches

Seminal vesicles covered by intact aponeurosis

Rectum

Prostate

Urethral catheter

Figure 9 : The dissection is pursued posteriorly and laterally, preserving the lateral pelvic fascia on one or both sides when it is decided to preserve erection, provided there is no oncological risk. Haemostasis is ensured by clips or fine Vicryl sutures. It is important to preserve the integrity of Denonvillier's fascia over the entire posterior surface of the prostate and seminal vesicles.

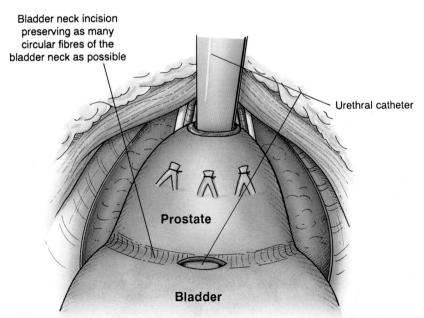

Bladder neck incision preserving as many circular fibres of the bladder neck as possible

Urethral catheter

Prostate

Bladder

Figure 10 : The anterior surface of the bladder neck is incised while attempting to preserve as many circular fibres as possible.

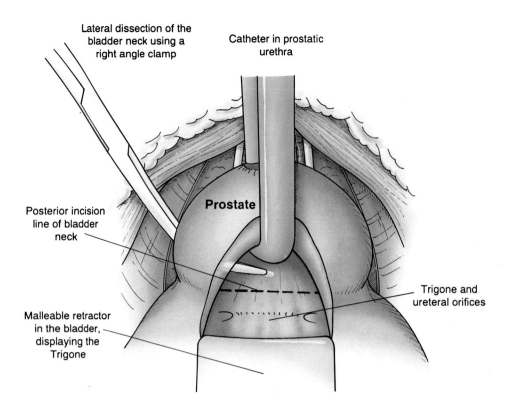

Lateral dissection of the bladder neck using a right angle clamp

Catheter in prostatic urethra

Prostate

Posterior incision line of bladder neck

Trigone and ureteral orifices

Malleable retractor in the bladder, displaying the Trigone

Figure 11 : Once the bladder neck is open, the ureteral orifices are located and incision of the posterior wall of the bladder neck can be done safely.

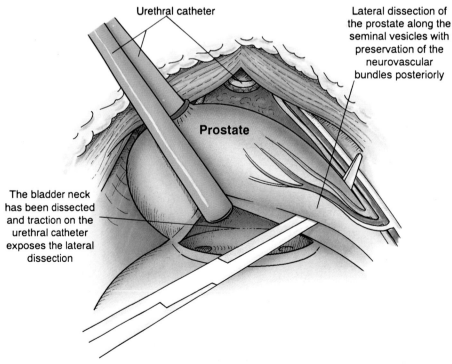

Urethral catheter

Lateral dissection of the prostate along the seminal vesicles with preservation of the neurovascular bundles posteriorly

Prostate

The bladder neck has been dissected and traction on the urethral catheter exposes the lateral dissection

Figure 12 : Gentle traction on the urethral catheter exposes the lateral dissection of the prostate and allows haemostasis of the last vascular pedicles on the lateral surfaces of the seminal vesicles. The neurovascular bundles can be damaged during dissection of the top of the seminal vesicles. Release of the prostate is completed by section of the vasa deferentes in the midline using large clips.

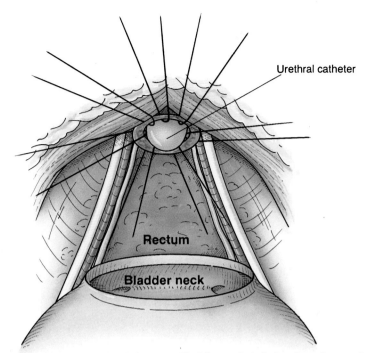

Urethral catheter

Rectum

Bladder neck

Figure 13 : Preparation of the so-called "parachute" direct vesico urethral anastomosis: some 10 3-O Vicryl stitches have been placed harmoniously around the urethra :

- in the anterior layer, the stitches take a strong bite on the pre-urethral fascia. The striated fibers of the external sphincter will be included in the anastomosis.

- in the posterior layer, the stitches take hold of Denonvillier's fascia, which make this posterior layer stronger.

- the stitches on both lateral angles stay away from the neurovascular bundles, to decrease the risk of postoperative impotence.

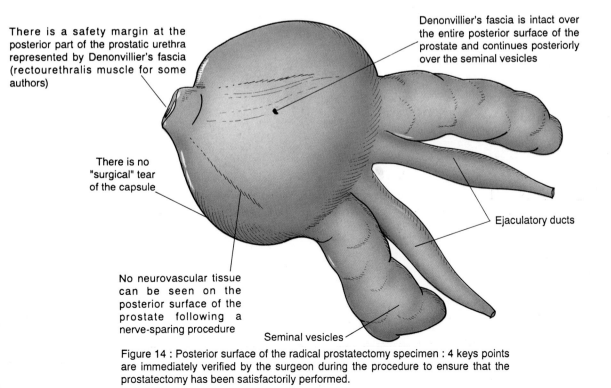

There is a safety margin at the posterior part of the prostatic urethra represented by Denonvillier's fascia (rectourethralis muscle for some authors)

Denonvillier's fascia is intact over the entire posterior surface of the prostate and continues posteriorly over the seminal vesicles

There is no "surgical" tear of the capsule

Ejaculatory ducts

No neurovascular tissue can be seen on the posterior surface of the prostate following a nerve-sparing procedure

Seminal vesicles

Figure 14 : Posterior surface of the radical prostatectomy specimen : 4 keys points are immediately verified by the surgeon during the procedure to ensure that the prostatectomy has been satisfactorily performed.

Does "anatomical" radical prostatectomy ensure satisfactory local control ?

R. Morton, M. Steiner and P. Walsh

J. Urol. 145, 1197 (1991)

Based on a precise knowledge of pelvic anatomy, particularly the dorsal vein complex and cavernous nerves, we have developed and used, since 1982, a precise operative technique in 586 patients with stage T1 (A) and T2 (B) prostatic cancer (with a follow-up of 1 to 8 years). This technique allows preservation of erection in 50 to 70% of cases and, in particular, allows a much more controlled dissection in order to ensure a better quality tumour resection, a decisive criterion which can only be assessed by regular evaluation of the results obtained over time.

1. What is the status of the patients after 5 years ?

The total recurrence rate was 11% with 4% of isolated local recurrences, 2% associated with distant metastases and 5% of isolated metastases (Table 1). Three patients died with or from cancer and 4 died without cancer.

Much less favourable results were observed when the margins were positive on pathological examination of the specimen (Table 2).

2. How do these results compare with those of other radical prostatectomy techniques ?

It is clear that the ideal yardstick for evaluation of efficacy of treatment of prostatic cancer is the *15-year survival*. However, an acceptable approximation is the *5-year recurrence rate,* as demonstrated by Catalona.

The various parameters can be compared to 8 major series in the literature. The local recurrence rate achieved with "anatomical" radical prostatectomy are as good and often better than those obtained by more extensive and less precise techniques (Table 2).

However, randomized studies with 15 year follow-up will be necessary to confirm the equality or superiority of "anatomical" prostatectomy.

Table 1. 5-Year status of 586 patients following radical prostatectomy based on preoperative clinical stage

Clinical Stage	No.	Local Recurrence	Distant Metastases		Elevated PSA	
			Alone	With Local Recurrence	Actuarial Analysis	Direct Analysis
A1	27	0	0	0	0	0
A2	59	7	5	2	4	5
B1N	98	0	4	0	7	7
B1	280	4	2	2	10	14
B2	122	8	12	7	40	16

Actuarial Status at 5 Yrs.

Table 2. Local recurrence without distant metastases following radical prostatectomy.

Reference	Stage		% Local Recurrence		
	Clinical	Pathological	5 Yrs.	10 Yrs.	15 Yrs.
Culp	B1				15*
Jewett		Neg. capsule			10
		Pos. capsule			33
Myers and Fleming †		Neg. capsule	8	10	
		Pos. capsule (±seminal vesicles)	20	45	
		Neg. seminal vesicles	5	12	12
		Pos. seminal vesicles	22	45	45
Middleton	A2		0		
	B1		6		
	B2		6		
Gibbons et al		Pos. capsule		25*	
		Pos. margin		17	
		Pos. seminal vesicles		44	
Anscher and Prosnitz		Neg. capsule	26‡		
		Pos. capsule	25		
		Neg. seminal vesicles	22		
		Pos. seminal vesicles	27		
		Neg. margin	20		
		Pos. margin	31		
Oesterling et al	B1N			0§	
	B1			25	
	B2			20	
		Neg. capsule		25	
		Pos. capsule (±seminal vesicles)		17	
Walsh et al	B1		7		
		Neg. capsule	10		
		Pos. capsule	10		
		Pos. seminal vesicles	0		
Blute et al		Neg. capsule	9‡		22

* Mean followup 10 years.
† 21% received adjuvant therapy.
‡ Mean followup 6 years.
§ Mean followup 9 years.

Does temporary occlusion of the hypogastric arteries resolve the problems of perioperative blood loss in radical prostatectomy ?

L. Kavoussi et al.
J. Urol. 146, 362 (1991)

For a long time, total prostatectomy had a reputation of being a haemorrhagic operation and various solutions have been proposed to control this blood loss, as better control is associated with the following advantages :

◆ decreased operative and anaesthetic trauma,

◆ decreased transfusion risk (HBs, HIV),

◆ clearer operating field, allowing better preservation of vital structures (continence, erection) and more satisfactory tumour resection.

P.C. Walsh et al. described controlled ligation of the deep dorsal vein and Santorini's plexus which greatly improved the resection from all of the above points of view.

They subsequently proposed temporary occlusion of the hypogastric arteries by 2 bulldog clamps immediately after lymph node dissection and reported a 40% decrease in transfusion requirements.

Lastly, they showed that the use of regional anaesthesia decreased blood loss by another 30%.

Knowing from personal experience the difficulty of interpreting the variation in blood losses in a retrospective series of patients (they compared 13 initial patients without clamping with a later series of 93 patients with clamping), we conducted this randomized study of 130 radical prostatectomies with and without temporary occlusion of the hypogastric arteries. We also compared 116 patients undergoing general anaesthesia with 15 operated under regional anaesthesia (non-randomized).

◆ *1* : clamping *did not decrease operative blood loss,* transfusion requirements or the drop of the haematocrit (Figure 1).

◆ *2* : regional anaesthesia did not affect these parameters either.

◆ *3* : the use of *three units of autologous blood* would have *eliminated the need for transfusion in 82% of patients*.

◆ *4 :* one must be very cautious when estimating operative blood losses, as the parameters measured can easily be altered by the proportion of urine mixed in the blood in the operating field and by the changing habits of anaesthetists concerning the amount of crystalloids administered routinely, the haematocrit below which transfusion is indicated and the haematocrit at which they consider that the operation should be terminated.

BLOOD LOSS

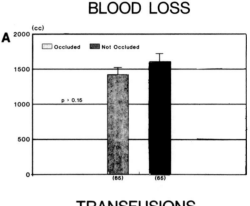
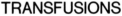

TRANSFUSIONS

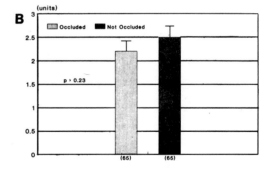

CHANGE IN HEMATOCRIT

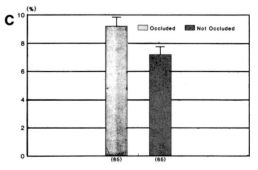

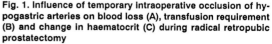

Fig. 1. Influence of temporary intraoperative occlusion of hypogastric arteries on blood loss (A), transfusion requirement (B) and change in haematocrit (C) during radical retropubic prostatectomy

Place of antegrade radical prostatectomy

J.A. Petros and W.J. Catalona
J. Urol. 145, 994 (1991)

When dissection is difficult during radical prostatectomy with nerve-sparing procedures, the operator is faced with a dilemma : should the cancer be considered to be unresectable or should the operation be continued by means of a different technique adapted to this particular situation ?

We opted for this second solution. Between May 1985 and November 1989, we performed 335 radical prostatectomies for cancer clinically confined to the prostate and in 30 cases we found the prostate to be adherent to the periprostatic tissues making the standard operation impossible. In these cases, we continued the operation via an *antegrade approach*. The first stage in the operation consisted of bladder neck incision followed by release of the seminal vesicles. At this stage, it was determined whether the infiltration was *inflammatory* (history of resection, multiple biopsies, prostatitis and/or diffuse, symmetrical appearance of the infiltration), in which case we preserved the neurovascular bundles. When the infiltration appeared to be due to *tumour* (gross appearance, frankly localized and unilateral process, particularly on the side of the lesion detected on rectal examination), the neurovascular bundles were sacrificed. The retroprostatic dissection, urethral section and vesicourethral anastomosis were then performed

1. What were our results in terms of the quality of tumour resection and negative margins? and how do these results compare with those of the 305 standard retrograde prostatectomies ?

The surgical margins were positive in 14 of the 30 antegrade prostatectomies (47%) versus 128 of the 305 retrograde prostatectomies (42%), i.e. equivalent rates with the two techniques. Table 1 shows the preoperative stage [T2b (B2) in 71% of cases], and sites of extension. Neurovascular bundles were spared unilaterally in 11 out of 14 cases and bilaterally in 1 cases).

A total of 12 cases undergoing a unilateral or bilateral nerve-sparing procedure were therefore found to have pathological stage pT3 (C) disease, with positive lateral margins in 9 cases, which confirms, in our opinion, the great difficulty of determining whether or not the neurovascular bundles are invaded at operation.

2. Potency was preserved to a similar degree by the two techniques when at least one neurovascular bundle was preserved.

3. Similarly, urinary continence was as good as with the standard operation.

In conclusion: These results suggest that the antegrade approach to radical retropubic prostatectomy can achieve rates of postoperative potency and urinary continence similar to those of the retrograde approach. Using an antegrade approach when the normal periprostatic tissue planes are obliterated makes an otherwise difficult dissection proceed smoothly. While the overall likelihood of complete tumour excision is not adversely affected, there is a tendency toward positive lateral margins.

We believe that if the antegrade approach is adopted because of periprostatic fibrosis, wide excision of the neurovascular bundles should be done to minimize the incidence of positive lateral surgical margins.

Table 1. Site (s) of extraprostatic extension in patients with pathological stage C (pT3) disease.

Pt. No.	Clinical Stage	Site(s) of Extension
1	B2	Lat., posterior
2	B2	Urethra
3	B2	Lat.
4	B1	Lat., posterior
5	B2	Lat., seminal vesicle
6	A2	Lat.
7	B2	Lat., seminal vesicle, urethra
8	B2	Lat., urethra
9	A2	Lat., bladder neck
10	B2	Post., urethra
11	B2	Bladder neck
12	B2	Lat.
13	B2	Lat.
14	B1	Apex, bladder neck

Does radical prostatectomy for incidental stage T1 (A) cancer detected on TUR or open excision of BPH differ from the standard technique ?

M. Bressel

in : Incidental carcinoma of the prostate, Springer
Verlag, Berlin, Heidelberg, 1991, 209-215.

Our experience of radical prostatectomy in stage T1(A) disease (based on 40 operations performed between May 1970 and November 1989 out of a total of 774 radical prostatectomies for cancer) revealed 2 essential features at this stage :

1. After resection, the **bladder neck is much wider** than during primary radical prostatectomy, which raises the technical problem of adapting the urethra to this wide bladder neck at the time of the anastomosis, with a potential increased risk of incontinence and stricture.

2. **Adhesions** are obviously present in the operative field, which may make dissection longer, more difficult and potentially less precise. P.C. Walsh has clearly shown that the precision of dissection is a very important factor in the quality of the postoperative functional results.

The operation is generally performed according to the usual stages, apart from the following specific features:

1. **Dissection of the apical region** may be more difficult and should therefore be performed very carefully.

2. The **plane between the two layers of Denonvillier's fascia** is often less well defined and must be clearly exposed. In particular, if the rectal muscle fibers are visible, the correct layer for dissection has not been reached.

3. **Reconstruction of the bladder neck** is a very important part of the operation. Firstly, during anterior dissection of the seminal vesicles, the surgeon presses his index finger between the ejaculatory ducts, against the tissue at the bladder-prostate junction and cuts the tissue raised in this way by scissors, in order to reach the bladder neck rather than the base of the trigone (Figure 1).

In any case, the bladder neck is generally too wide. We insert a 22 F Tiemann catheter into the wide bladder neck opening and perform two small incisions underneath this catheter (Figure 2). Using Vicryl sutures, a bladder outlet tube is made at the future site of anastomosis, which we complete by drawing the edges of the bladder together by means of three Z purse string sutures, resulting in an additional support for the base of the bladder. The bladder is then filled with 200 cc of water; no fluid should leak from the bladder neck, but pressing the bladder with the finger generates a stream of water. To lessen the strain on the anastomosis, two lateral relief sutures are placed from the base of the bladder to the pelvic floor muscles, lateral to the neurovascular bundles.

The wound is drained by 3 Redon suction drainages.

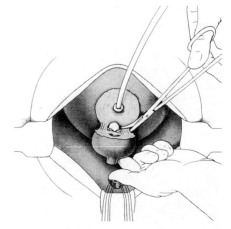

Fig. 1. In order to find the correct layer between the base of bladder and the seminal vesicles, the dissection follows the surgeon's fingertip, which is inserted between the ejaculatory ducts up to the 6 o'clock position of the bladder neck.

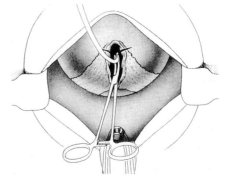

Fig. 2. Reconstruction of the wide bladder neck. A 22 F Tiemann catheter armed with a Mixter clamp is introduced. The 6 o'clock point of the new bladder outlet is determined. A 2 cm vertical incision is made on both sides through the whole bladder wall, in order to form a small flap. Before taking this step it is useful to insert two catgut stitches at the 1 and 11 o'clock position.

Technical nuances and surgical results of radical retropubic prostatectomy in 150 patients

Paul Lange and Pratap Reddy.

J. Urol. 138, 348 (1987)

We report here several key observations that we have made in the course of performing 150 radical prostatectomies for prostatic carcinoma, which we think can make this operation easier to perform, hence rendering it safer for the patient as well as diminishing the rate of undesirable events and complications. Some of these pointers are fairly straightforward, yet deserve reporting because of their usefulness.

1. Patient positioning

a) extension of the lumbar spine: like many surgeons, we believe it is important to position the patient with a slight extension of the lumbar spine by "breaking" the table, when possible, or by placing a rolled blanket under the sacrum. This, combined with a Trendelenburg or reversed Trendelenburg tilt of the table, as appropriate, can greatly improve visualisation into the deep pelvis.

b) position of the legs: this is, in our opinion, a most important nuance. By putting the patient in a modified lithotomy position, with legs apart by approximately 35 degrees, a sponge stick can be used at crucial points during the operation to exert a cephalad pressure on the perineum, thus bringing the urogenital diaphragm into better view within the pelvis to control bleeding and to perform the vesico-urethral anastomosis (Figure 1). It is not uncommon for the urogenital diaphragm to extend 3 to 5 cm into the pelvis, converting a potentially difficult suture placement for haemostasis or for the anastomosis into a relatively easy and safe surgical manoeuvre. To avoid pressure injuries to the calves during the operation, we have developed special stirrups, which hold them in a sort of hammock: to further reduce the risk of deep vein thrombosis, we also use sequential pneumatic leg compression devices.

2. Management of the dorsal vein complex

a) pubo prostatic ligaments should be taken cautiously, in small increments, using palpation rather than vision to determine if sufficient fibrous attachment remains to justify pursuing this manoeuvre.

b) suture ligature of the complex: after tying a ligature around it as described by Reiner and Walsh, we find it safer to pass a suture through it with a needle. The suture is then passed through the space provided by the right angle clamp and tied to form a suture ligature of the area.

c) wedge pubectomy: in cases where a good exposure is difficult to obtain, we cut a trapezoidal wedge of pubis, 3 by 5 cm. This seemingly insignificant pubectomy can enhance visualization considerably. In the 49 patients in which we performed it, we have had only one case of suprapubic pain lasting for 6 months.

d) temporary haemostasis of the perineal field: when suture ligature of remaining bleeding veins with 5/8 circle 2-0 chromic sutures does not provide a fully satisfactory haemostasis, we have used (once the urethra has been transected and a preliminary space has been developed between the prostate and the rectum) a Foley catheter, its balloon inflated to 5 cc and a sponge wrapped under the balloon, and exerted a light traction on it. It is helpful to cut off the tip of the catheter to make it less obtrusive.

3. Vesico-urethral anastomosis

a) we do not feel it is useful to place the sutures at the time of transection of the prostato-urethal junction.

b) we attempt to preserve the circular fibers of the bladder neck to insure a smooth circular configuration of about 26F.

4. Patient selection

We have not found added difficulties in cases operated after a TURP or an open prostatectomy. We usually allow a two week interval bewween the initial operation and the radical prostatectomy.

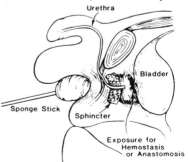

Figure 1. Application of appropriate pressure in the perineum allows for better exposure.

Complications of Radical Prostatectomy

F. Sole Balcells

Fundation Puigvert, Barcelona, Spain

The bases for this report are the 79 Radical Prostatectomies we have done at the Fundacion Puigvert between April of 1985 and August of 1991 and a discussion of the experience gained from major international series.

Altogether our patients were 2 stage T1a, 9 T1b, 62 T2 and 6 T3, which turned out on final pathological examination to be 4 pT0, 23 pT2, 45 pT3 and 7 patients with positive nodes (N+).

Our *initial complication rate* was a low 16% (vesico-cutaneous fistula, lymphocele, wound infection and hematoma, all healed with 3 re-operations).

Our *long term local complication rate* was 24.2%, with stress incontinence in 15.5%, impotence in 39.4% and stenosis at the anastomotic site in 17.5% (which resolved with 16 direct vision urethrotomies in 14 patients).

At the end of the follow up (mean 34 months) *87.3%* of the patients were *alive disease free, 5.6% alive with disease* and *1.3% dead of disease.*

Comparing our own series with others, it is obvious that the complications of radical prostatectomy, general and local, are a *complex function* of the status of the patient (general condition and associated illnesses), the prostatic neoplastic disease (stage, grade, cancer volume, previous interventions on the prostate...) and the skill and experience of the surgeon (Table 1).

More important to discuss than the *non specific complications* (thromboembolism, infection, lymphoceles...) are *local delayed complications* : incontinence, impotence, stricture at the anastomotic site and cancer recurrences.

1. Post-prostatectomy incontinence

This complication is variously reported (Table 2). It is accepted by most authors to be extremly high in the first month (100% for P. Lange), but only 53% at 3 months and 8% at two years, displaying a clear *trend for improvement with time* (C. Brendler and P.C.Walsh). It has not been possible to pinpoint a precise parameter in those patients that remain incontinent. In some series, an anatomical, nerve-sparing operation seems associated with a higher early continence rate (O'Donnel) while others have reported a higher rate following preoperative androgenic blockade (Schulman) . A technical point seems worth attention which was raised by P.C. Walsh: recognising that the *external sphincter* extends anteriorly where it is an *integral part of the dorsal vein complex,* he recommends that one should suture tie it in a *transverse* fashion at the time of taking the dorsal vein so that it will *lie anteriorly to the anastomosis and become integrated to it.* With this technical modification, he has been able to bring his 3 month continence rate up to 73%, from 47% previously.

In an effort to improve on the continence rate, some authors (Presti, Walsh) have

Table 1 : The post-radical prostatectomy complications are related to:

- patient age
- performance status, associated illnesses
- grade and tumour stage
- volume of the tumour
- previous treatments (TUR)
- surgeon's experience
- surgical technique

Table 2 : Urinary continence post-radical prostatectomy :

Incontinence : 0.5-11%, depending upon the definition of incontinence :
- no case of incontinence in 50 R/P (Lange)
- 98% continence in 192 R/P at 6 months (Catalona)

at 3 m - 47%	8% stress inc.	in 600 R/P
at 12 m - 89%	0% total inc.	(WALSH)
at 24 m - 92%		

Table 3 : How to avoid urinary incontinence after R/P ?

- Urethro-vesical anastomosis with fixation of the external sphincter to the deep venous complex (the external sphincter is attached to the bladder neck)
- Bladder outlet tubularization (tennis-racket)
- Eversion of the bladder-mucosa at the bladder outlet.

Table 4 : Anastomotic urethro-vesical stricture.

Incidence : 9.6% - 17.7%
How to avoid strictures ?
- meticulous operative haemostasis
- careful approximation of bladder mucosa over bladder neck section
- precise mucosa to mucosa anastomosis of bladder neck to urethra

funnelized the distal bladder above the bladder neck, creating a sort of neourethra, which increased the total length of the urethra, and observed a higher incontinence rate when that length could not be increased to about 2.5 cm (Table 3)

2. Stricture at the anastomotic site

This complication has been reported in approximately 10% of cases in several major series. Its incidence can be reduced (Table 4) by:

- careful approximation of the bladder mucosa over the muscular edge of the cut section of the bladder neck,

- approximating the urethra and bladder neck strictly mucosa to mucosa,

- ensuring meticulous haemostasis, as postoperative perianastomotic haematomas tend to induce fibrosis, as does urine leakage through the anastomosis.

It is recommended, in case of stricture, to cut it with a cold knife, as use of the hot knife has been associated with post procedure incontinence.

3. Sexual function

The anatomical approach to nerve-sparing prostatectomy has made the operation a much more valuable therapeutic option.

W. Catalona (Table 5) reports a potency rate of 63% in bilateral bundle preservation and 39% in case of unilateral sacrifice of the bundle on the side of the lesion. P.C. Walsh reports respectively an 76% and 63% potency rate in bilateral and unilateral preservation, with **results being much better in patients under age 50**. One should stress, however, that the **primary goal of this operation is cancer control** : potency sparing should not be attempted if it would compromise in any way this primary goal.

4. Local and distant failures

In discussing outcome of prostatectomy, it is important to distinguish the cases which, on final pathological analysis of the whole prostate specimen, are:

Table 5 : Sexual potency after radical prostatectomy.

CATALONA : 112 cases
with neuro-vascular preservation :
  • bilateral - 63% potent
  • unilateral - 39% potent
WALSH : 503 cases
with neuro-vascular preservation :
  • bilateral   - 76% potent
  • unilateral - 63% potent
but : great importance of age :
  • < 50 years - 91%
  • > 75 years - 25%

Table 6 : Local failure at 5 years is closely related to the limits of cancer in the specimen. (Results from Walsh)

	Local rec.	Mets	↗PSA
Organ confined	2%	1%	3%
Specimen confined	8%	1%	16%
Positive margins	8%	19%	41%

Table 7 : Treatment of capsular penetration and/or positive margins.

Some authors : no treatment (same survival with or without capsular penetration)
  • 85% tumour free at 5 years
  • 70% tumour free at 10 years (FARROW)
Others : adjuvant radiotherapy
  • diminishes risk of local failure : 4.1% (DOUCHEZ)
  • increases interval free of disease (AUSCHER)
  • but does not modify survival rate (PAULSON)

◆ *organ confined*

◆ *specimen confined* (infiltration of the capsule, but negative surgical margin),

◆ or have *positive margins*, which carry a different long-term prognosis, with a local recurrence rate of 2%, 8% and 8% respectively and metastases in 1%, 1%, 19% respectively, at 5 years in a report by Walsh (Table 6). *Preoperative prediction of the final pathological findings as stratified above is not fully reliable.* PSA and PAP values or transrectal ultrasound are of little value in the individual patient. Certainly the risk of positive margins increases with cancer volume, but preoperative volume measurement, even with TRUS, is not entirely reproducible, and the cut-off value has been estimated differently by various authors. When a nerve-sparing prostatectomy is performed, P.C. Walsh and J. Epstein have been able to show that positive margins at the sole site of the preserved bundle were highly unusual.

Once positivity of margins has been established, there is no consensus on what if any adjuvant treatment should be offered.

a) Watchful waiting has been recommended by those who have not observed a decrease in overall survival as compared to that of patients with negative margins on the specimen.

b) Radiation therapy seems to decrease the incidence of local recurrence or elevation of PSA, but long-term comparative studies are lacking to define its impact on survival. A study by Paulson points to the absence of benefit from radiation therapy in this setting, yet one might argue that it may help *decrease the incidence of local recurrences and increase the disease free interval.*

c) A similar controversy exists regarding *hormonal manipulation* in cases of positive margins, persistent elevation of PSA after radical prostatectomy, or positive TRUS-guided biopsies of the anastomotic site.

◆ *Positive lymph nodes*

A more detailed discussion of this issue will be conducted elsewhere. We will only mention here that P.C. Walsh and J. de Kernion (the latter in a randomized study) found *no increased survival in patients receiving early hormonal manipulation,* but only an increase in disease free interval.

The management of rectal injury during radical retropubic prostatectomy

R. Neil Borland and P.C. Walsh.

J. Urol. 147, 905 (1991)

The risk of rectal injury during radical prostatectomy has been a major concern to urologists performing this operation leading to the widespread use of full preoperative bowel preparation and antibiotics and to the recommendation of proximal fecal diversion if an injury does occur. We reviewed the 10 rectal injuries that occurred in the course of 1000 radical prostatectomies for localised disease in *non irradiated patients*.

All injuries were full thickness rectal lacerations less than 2 cm long. No patient had received preoperative antibiotics, and only a simple enema had been used for bowel preparation. Nine of the 10 injuries occurred *during the division of the posterior aspect of the striated urethral sphincter at a point where there was fibrosis and fixation to the rectum*. One of the 10 injuries was caused during *wide excision of a neuro-vascular bundle*.

In all other patients, the injury was recognized during the operation. In these cases, the radical prostatectomy was completed, the bladder neck reconstructed and the anastomotic sutures placed. At that point, the *anal sphincter was dilated* to 3 fingerbreadths by the assistant. With the added exposure of the assistant's finger in the rectum, the injury was closed with an inner layer of continuous 2-0 chromic and an outer layer of interrupted 2-0 silk Lambert stitches. A small peritoneal opening was made above the bladder and a properly sized omental pedicle was constructed: if a long pedicle was needed, the omentum was separated from the colon and off the stomach as described by Turner-Warwick. It was then passed through another small peritoneal opening between the rectum and bladder and was tacked down with interrupted 2-0 chromic sutures so as to cover the area of repair completely. The procedure was then completed as usual, with suction drains placed on both paravesical spaces. Broad spectrum antibiotics were given for 7 to 14 days. Nasogastric suction was not used. Bowel softeners and mineral oil were used for 6 weeks.

In *one case*, the injury was diagnosed on *postoperative day 2 with* the development of fever and fecaluria, immediate re-exploration was conducted: the urethrovesical anastomosis was taken down to reveal the source of the leakage (if need be, a rectal finger probing gently can help identify the lesion). After the lesion was repaired as described above and the urethro vesical anastomosis completed, a *diverting loop sigmoidostomy* was constructed in the left lower quadrant. The *colostomy was taken down 3 months later.*

With this management, all injuries healed uneventfully.

The experience gained with these patients highlights several key principles:

◆ opposing suture lines should be avoided.

◆ *interposition of healthy tissues* between urinary and gastrointestnal tract is very important. *An omental pedicle* is ideally suited to promote uneventful healing, with the added advantage here of allowing a good urodynamic mobility.

◆ *a full bowel preparation or preoperative antibiotics are not necessary* before radical prostatectomy in non irradiated patients

◆ *a diverting colostomy is indicated only in case of delayed diagnosis*, and certainly in patients *irradiated preoperatvely* or with otherwise compromised healing potential.

In summary, primary repair of rectal injury with the greater omentum and without a diverting colostomy is safe, effective and associated with minimal patient morbidity.

Radical prostatectomy and preservation of potency : has the controversy been resolved?

D. Quinlan, J. Epstein, B. Carter, P. Walsh
J. Urol. 145, 998 (1991)

The understanding of the anatomy of the prostate, cavernous nerves and dorsal vein complex has led to preservation of the neurovascular bundles allowing the postoperative preservation of sexual function.

However, very rapidly, two basic questions were raised concerning this procedure :

◆ *what rate of preservation of erection could be realistically announced to patients and for each individual patient?*

◆ *and what was the cancer risk to the patient in this operation which appeared to pass very close to the malignant organ?*

In reality, far from compromising the resection, this technique, when it is indicated, allows a more complete excision to be performed, particularly of the neurovascular bundles themselves, than that achieved by standard procedures.

We have now performed this operation in more than 600 cases and the best way to answer these questions was to review these case records from these two points of view. We analysed 503 patients who reported sexual activity prior to the operation and who were followed for at least 18 months.

1. Does preservation of one or both cavernous nerves increase the cancer risk?

Of the 492 patients with clinical stage T1(A) or T2 (B) disease in this series, *49 had positive margins* (10%, which is in the same range as in series without nerve-sparing), but *only 9 (2%) of these patients had positive margins in the area of the preserved neurovascular bundle* (excision of the second neurovascular bundle would have prevented this positivity in only one case) and none of these 9 patients have developed a local recurrence to date.

We believe that extracapsular extension is palpable during the operation in the form of induration. In such cases, total resection of the tumour should ob-

viously take priority, even if one or both neurovascular bundles must be deliberately sacrificed. A high rate of postoperative potency can be achieved even after preservation of a single neurovascular bundle.

2. When should the neurovascular bundles not be preserved?

a) Preoperative decision :

. patient with no real sexual activity

. invasion of the lateral groove (stage T3-T4)

b) Intraoperative decision :

. palpable extraprostatic extension

. fixation of the neurovascular bundle

. caution is advised in the case of apical tumours due to the high risk of extracapsular extension.

3. What sexual potency preservation rate can be announced to the patient and what are the factors which influence the return of sexual function ?

a) Our overall postoperative potency rate in this series was 68%.

b) Age : potency was preserved in men: (Figure 1)

less than 50 years old	90%
50 to 59 years old	75%
60 to 69 years old	58%
over 70 years old	25%.

c) The clinical stage is very important : obviously more advanced stages are closely correlated with wider excision with 85 to 100% potency for stage T1(A) and 56 to 64% for stage T2 (B) (Table 1).

d) The pathological stage : the risk of postoperative impotence is doubled in the case of pathological stage pT3 disease.

e) Surgical technique : the postoperative potency rate was :

◆ preservation of the two neurovascular bundles: 76%

◆ preservation of one neurovascular bundle and partial preservation of the other: 68%

◆ preservation of a single neurovascular bundle : 63%

◆ sacrifice of both neurovascular bundles: 0%

f) Potency is recovered more rapidly when the two neurovascular bundles have been preserved.

In conclusion, an "anatomical" technique in correctly selected patients allows preservation of potency in a very significant proportion of cases without compromising the quality of cancer resection.

Table 1. Influence of clinical stage and operative technique on return of sexual function.

Age (yrs.)	Neurovascular Bundles*	Clinical Stage (% potent postop.)				
		A1	B1N	B1	A2	B2
<50	++	100	90.9	92.8	100	50
	+±	100	—	100	—	—
	+0	—	—	75	—	100
50–59	++	85.7	95.1	80.0	64.3	54.5
	+±	100	60.0	79.2	80.0	55.5
	+0	100	100	58.8	100	54.1
60–69	++	80	75	70.5	69.2	57.1
	+±	—	80	46.2	40	50
	+0	—	100	36.4	0	65
>70	++	—	0	40	0	—
	+±	—	—	50	—	—
	+0	—	—	—	—	0
All ages	++	85	85.9	75.7	65.5	55.5
	+±	100	70.0	64.3	60.0	52.9
	+0	100	100	48.8	75	63.5

* ++, Preservation neurovascular bundles bilaterally; +±, partial excision of 1 neurovascular bundle; +0, wide excision of 1 neurovascular bundle.

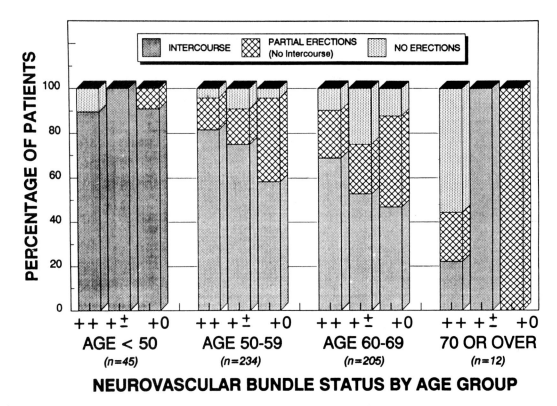

Figure 1. Influence of age and surgical technique on return of sexual function after radical prostatectomy. Ther was only 1 patient in + ± and +o groups in patients 70 or more years old.

Urinary continence following radical anatomical prostatectomy

C.B. Brendler, R.A. Morton, M.S. Steiner
and P.C. Walsh

Urol. Cl. Nth. Am. 17, 679 (1990)

One of the most dreaded complications of radical prostatectomy is urinary incontinence. The *anatomical approach* to this operation has resulted in *several modifications in surgical technique* to reduce the incidence of this complication:

1. techniques providing a *bloodless field* with excellent exposure.

2. precise apical dissection to *avoid injury to the pelvic floor musculature and preservation of the putative autonomic branches* for the striated sphincter that course in the neurovascular bundles.

3. an *accurate sutured vesico-urethral anastomosis* with coaptation of the mucosal surfaces.

4. incorporation of the *sphincteric elements of the dorsal vein complex* into the anastomosis: this is a very important new technical nuance that results from the recognition that the external sphincter has a *vertical extension that wraps around the membranous urethra and the prostate.* Its anterior part is integrated into the dorsal vein complex. After transection, this structure should be *oversewn horizontally* using 2-0 chromic catgut. This manoeuvre forms an anterior hood of tissue that will be helpful in decreasing the risk both of incontinence and of stricture formation.

5. identification and sharp division of the *posterior component of the striated sphincter* during the separation of the posterior aspect of the prostate from the rectum.

We reviewed 600 radical prostatectomies performed by one of us (P.C.W.) of which 86 where stage T1 (A), 500 T2 (B) and 14 T3 (C).

Complete urinary continence was achieved in 92%. *Stress incontinence* was present in 8%. Six per cent wore one or less pad per day. Thus, *98% of the patients were either dry or wore at most one pad per day.* No patient was totally incontinent, but two have undergone the placement of an *artificial sphincter*, because of severe stress incontinence. At 3 months 47% were dry, at 6 months 75%, at 9 months 82%, at 12 months 89% and at 2 years 92%.

The only factor that influenced long-term continence was age. Urinary continence returned in 100% of men less than 40 years of age, and 86% of men aged 70-76 years.

Prior transurethral resection of the prostate, pathologic stage, preservation or wide excision of one or both neurovascular bundles and prostate weight had no influence on postoperative continence.

In reviewing the literature, urinary continence following radical prostatectomy varies between 63 and 93%, with 0-35% experiencing stress incontinence and 0-17% of patients complaining of total urinary incontinence. Contrary to our observation, prior TURP had an adverse effect on the recovery of continence.

Meticulous attention to surgical technique helps to achieve higher rates of continence.

Radical perineal prostatectomy

I. INTRODUCTION

The potential development of *laparoscopic lymph node dissection* has led to a renewed interest in transperineal radical prostatectomy, as it can be performed *as a second operation when the definitive histological results of lymph node dissection are available*. Transperineal radical prostatectomy, which was initially the preferred approach for radical prostatectomy, has been replaced by the retropubic approach, which was considered to offer the great advantage of allowing evaluation of the lymph nodes via the same route. The place of transperineal radical prostatectomy therefore needs to be re-evaluated in the current context.

It is also generally accepted that radical prostatectomy performed *after transurethral resection and even more so after open prostatectomy* is often more difficult with poorer results in terms of urinary continence. By approaching the organ via a *previously untouched route*, transperineal radical prostatectomy may be especially indicated in this situation.

II. TECHNIQUE

P.B. Hudson

University of South Florida, Florida, USA

Particularly adapted to *obese patients* and those with a poorly developed perineal musculature, as is frequently the case in elderly patients, transperineal radical prostatectomy allows *as complete a resection as retropubic radical prostatectomy with less trauma, requiring less profound anaesthesia, causing less blood loss and allowing more precise anatomical reconstruction of urological structures.*

1. Is any particular preparation required?

Apart from the fact that, in the case of laparoscopic lymph node dissection, the definitive histological results should be available prior to the operation, the only precaution is to ensure that the intestine has been completely evacuated by enemas. *Three assistants* are required together with an instrument nurse to perform the operation under ideal conditions of safety. *Curved and straight prostatic retractors are essential.*

When installing the patient on the table, the *buttocks must be raised much higher* than for any other form of surgery so that the *perineum is perfectly horizontal, fa-*

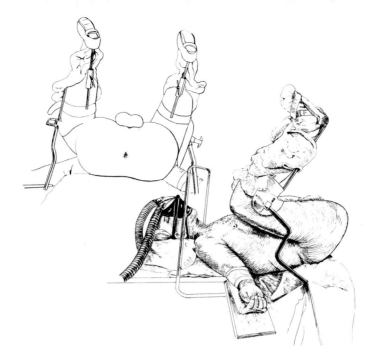

Figure 1. The lower section of the table is turned down in a vertical direction, and an instrument tray is affixed to this portion. The upper portion of the table is elevated at an angle of 30 degrees. The patient's position is maintained by the shoulder braces and by the pressure exerted on the foot by the stirrup mechanism. Note that the perineum is in an almost horizontal position. The upper extremity is extended at an angle that does not exceed 45 degrees with the long axis of the torso. Limitation of abduction in this way prevents temporary brachial palsy. Pronation of the arm also prevents brachial palsy.

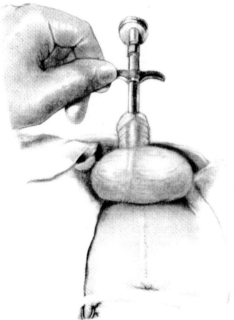

Figure 2. The curved urethral tractor has been inserted, rotated to determine that its tip is well within the lumen of the bladder, and the blades have been opened by clockwise rotation of the knob. This instrument is held firmly by the crosspiece. The assistant's wrist should rest upon the patient's thigh.

Subcutaneous anal sphincter

Figure 3. The double dotted lines indicate the position of the subcutaneous anal sphincter. Topically, this is indicated by wrinkling or puckering of the skin external to the mucocutaneous junction.

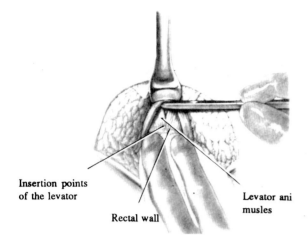

Insertion points
of the levator

Rectal wall

Levator ani
musles

Figure 4. The middle and index fingers of the left hand are still used in preference to a posterior or rectal retractor. It is seen that the slight midline separation in the leaves of the levator ani muscles has come into view. Notice is also taken of the insertion points of the levator on each side as it fuses directly with the external longitudinal smooth muscle of the ventral rectal wall.

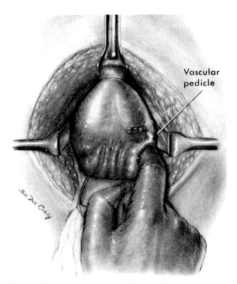

Vascular
pedicle

Figure 5. The curved urethral tractor has now been returned to the original position used for the preliminary dissection and biopsy. This brings the prostate prominently into the surgical wound. The left lateral aspect of the prostate is freed by blunt dissection. Close following of the anatomic capsule (anterior Denonvilliers' fascia) ensures avoidance of the lateral venous plexuses as the dissection proceeds ventrally around the gland. After both lateral aspects of the prostate are freed, the finger is swept toward the rectum until it encounters resistance from the vascular pedicle and fascial folds over the arteries and veins as they enter medially to supply the prostate and bladder neck regions. The vessels in this pedicle are derived mainly from branches of the inferior vesical artery.

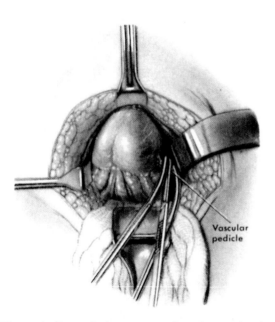

Vascular
pedicle

Figure 6. Curved clamps are placed completely across the left prostatic vascular pedicle, and the scalpel is used to divide it.

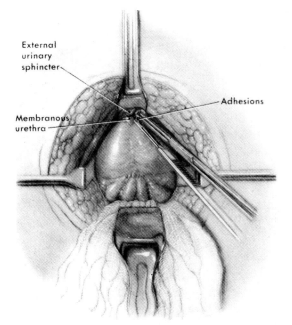

Figure 7. Remaining fibers of the external urinary sphincter are being pushed distally upon the membranous urethra. The scalpel is used to dissect any adhesions in order to avoid tearing, which ultimately would produce scar tissue and dysfunction.

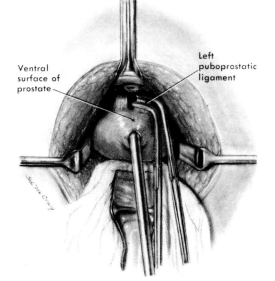

Figure 8. Right-angled hemostatic forceps have been applied to the patient's left puboprostatic ligament. The lower clamp should be placed as close as possible to the ventral surface of the prostate. In order to get exposure of this sort, light traction is exerted downward (toward the patient's coccyx). This places the puboprostatic ligaments on tension as they come clearly into view. Excessive traction is avoided to preclude tearing of the ventral surface of the prostate. Following division of these ligaments, the severed ends of each are secured with suture ligatures of OO chromic catgut.

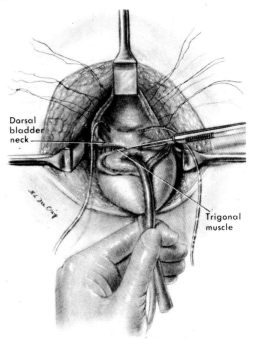

Figure 9. With a scalpel, the dorsal bladder neck is incised distal to the ureteral orifices. Preferably a margin of 1 cm is left between the cut edge of the orifices. These layers of muscle include the trigonal muscle as well as the detrusor fibers laterally.

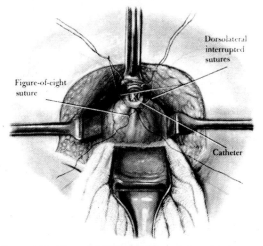

Figure 10. Two additional dorsolateral interrupted sutures have been placed and are ready to be tied. In addition, a figure-of-8-suture has been placed to complete the anastomosis. The knot on this suture is placed on the vesical rather than the membranous urethral side. The urethral bag catheter has been advanced into the bladder and inflated.

cing the ceiling of the operating room and protruding beyond the end of the table. The shoulders must be carefully protected because of the exaggerated Trendelenburg position of the table.

2. How is the operation performed ?

A perineal incision is performed to expose Denonvillier's fascia, the posterior layer of which is carefully retracted with the rectum. After dissecting around the prostate, the posterosuperior pedicles are isolated and sectioned. The sphincter is then directly visible and can be delicately reclined inferiorly before sectioning the urethra, avoiding any trauma responsible for fibrosis and subsequent incontinence. Lowsey's curved retractor is then replaced by the straight retractor, the anterior surface of the prostate is released and the puboprostatic ligaments are sectioned (*the dorsal vein complex is retracted from the zone of dissection in contrast with the retropubic approach*). The bladder neck is then sectioned and the seminal vesicles are released with excellent visual control. **The urethro-vesical anastomosis is also performed with remarkable exposure.**

3. Are any particular postoperative precautions required ?

No rectal temperature or rectal medications for a fortnight. The analgesic requirements are limited and no dressing is necessary after the first postoperative day. The perineal drain is removed on the third day, the patient is discharged from hospital on the 8th day and the catheter is removed on the 14th day.

The few problems which may be encountered during the postoperative period are no different from those following retropubic radical prostatectomy, apart from delayed healing or infection of the perineal incision due to the proximity of the anastomosis. In this case, the non-absorbable suture material should be left in place a little longer and the wound discharge should be cultured and treated by appropriate antibiotics. Warm baths can be administered twice a day. Rectal injuries or fistulae are not more frequent after this procedure and require the same preventive (meticulous dissection, intraoperative identification and immediate careful treatment) and corrective measures as retropubic radical prostatectomy (see section on complications below).

In conclusion : when performed for *appropriate indications* and according to a *rigorous technique*, transperineal radical prostatectomy should be considered very seriously in the treatment of prostatic cancer as an *oncologically effective, minimally traumatic operation allowing precise reconstruction.*

III. COMPLICATIONS

Perineal prostatectomy is a well tolerated procedure with reasonably few complications. *Precise strategies to deal with complications when they occur help keep a low morbidity to this operation.*

I. Inadvertent removal of indwelling urethral catheter

Accidental removal of the catheter after radical perineal prostatectomy should not be cause for alarm. Almost invariably the patient voids spontaneously. If spontaneous voiding does not occur, a considerable period of waiting is permissible.

If recatheterization is required following radical perineal prostatectomy, two courses are open to the surgeon. First, a *suprapubic tube* may be placed. Second, a *small-caliber indwelling urethral catheter* can be inserted *through a panendoscopic sheath*. This sheath should be introduced by direct vision panendoscopy of the anterior and membranous urethra *with extreme care* : It must be borne in mind that trauma to the line of anastomosis will cause separation of the bladder neck from the urethra, which is particularly undesirable following radical prostatectomy because it *predisposes to formation of a narrow, hard stricture in the space between the bladder neck and the urethra.*

2. Extravasation of urine

Urinary extravasation occurring after radical perineal prostatectomy is not uncommon during the first postoperative week. The drain lateral to the operative incision is simply left for a prolonged period of time, until all evidence of extravasation has ceased. If urinary extravasation occurs after the catheter has been removed on the fourteenth postoperative day, immediate recatheterization is indicated. The catheter is left indwelling for an additional 5 to 7 days, and the free drainage of extravasated urine is assured.

3. Improper drainage or occlusion of the indwelling catheter

After radical perineal prostatectomy, improper drainage from the indwelling urethral catheter is almost always the result of a *proximally angulated catheter tip.* The gradual withdrawal of fluid from the catheter bag, and **adjustment of the placement of the catheter** with constant observation to determine the point at which drainage is re-established, constitutes the preferred method of management. Gentle irrigation with 20 ml of irrigant is permissible. It is best not to use a piston-type syringe; undue hydrostatic pressure may cause leakage at the anastomotic line between the bladder neck and the membranous urethra.

4. Postoperative haemorrhage

Postoperative haemorrhage is almost never encountered. When it is, *one must suspect a blood dyscrasia* that was not disclosed during the routine preoperative evaluation.

Emergency haematological consultation is required. If bleeding from the wound is excessive, local haemostasis under infiltration anaesthesia should be undertaken promptly.

5. Urinary tract infection

Infection should be treated by changing the patient to a urinary antiseptic drug not previously employed immediately after the collection of an additional urine sample for culture and drug sensitivity testing. *The catheter is removed as soon as possible* in order to exclude the foreign body factor from the cycle of conditions that favor continuation of infection. Whenever there is inadequate drainage around the catheter, a smaller-caliber catheter is substituted.

6. Urinary fistula

Urinary fistula can be eradicated spontaneously by **prolonging the time of urethral catheter drainage**. Care should be taken to ascertain that the urinary drainage through the catheter is unobstructed.

7. Delayed wound healing and wound infection

The nonabsorbable sutures used to close the perineal skin are left for up to 2 weeks postoperatively. As soon as the catheter has been removed from the urethra, warm baths given twice daily will be beneficial. The apex of the lower lip of the incision may slough in an area of approximately 1 cm^2. This slough is almost invariably superficial, for it results from ischaemic necrosis of the small area supplied by arteries that have been divided as they traverse longitudinally the "central tendon" projection of the subcutaneous fibers of the external rectal sphincter.

8. Stress urinary incontinence

In the occasional patient with stress urinary incontinence or otherwise imperfect urinary control following perineal prostatectomy, the pre-existing obstruction will have required the development of very high intravesical pressures for micturition. There will be a period of reconditioning for the detrusor reflex arc while the bladder becomes accustomed to a reduced force of muscular contraction, both to initiate voiding and to serve as a level for "resting tone" of the detrusor. This fact **should be explained to the patient carefully**, and he should be prompted to continue the use of sphincteric voiding exercises.

9. Cystitis

Immediate therapy is limited to ordinary urinary antiseptics. This therapy is continued until the causative organism has been identified, which will permit rational antibiotic therapy.

Persistent or recurring cystitis suggests residual bladder urine, which makes cure most difficult. *Postvoiding urogram x-ray films should not be delayed* if cystitis is unresponsive to careful medicinal therapy.

In cases of highly viscous, purulent discharge, irrigation of the bladder with nonabsorbable antibiotics is most helpful.

In any event, therapy must be prompt and definitive if ascending pyelonephritis is to be prevented.

10. Fecal fistula

Fecal fistula is treated by **sterilization of the bowel**, using neomycin sulfate in a dosage of 1 gm per hour for four doses, followed by 1 gm every 4 hours. This program is followed for 72 hours and is then discontinued. Simultaneously with the start of the bowel sterilization program, the patient is placed on **parenteral feeding** with vitamin supplementation. The **rectal sphincter is dilated manually**, and a soft rectal tube is inserted for a distance of 14 cm. This tube is never irrigated but when occluded is replaced. The drainage by indwelling urethral catheter is continued until the fecal fistula is

closed. Warm baths, two or three times daily, in which the urethra and catheter are not submerged, assist in the healing process. Diligent adherence to this schedule prevents the formation of persistent fistulae.

11. Pyelonephritis

Parenchymal infection of the kidney is a disorder that requires prompt recognition and vigorous, persistent therapy. It may occur after all types of prostatic surgical operations. **A principal consideration is to rule out obstructive uropathy**. Either persistent residual urine or partial ureteral obstruction precludes eradication of pyelonephritis to the point of nonrecurrence.

Therefore, *intravenous urography* with a postvoiding film is required before a second course of drug therapy is instituted or whenever the first course fails.

12. Ureteral occlusion

Partial or complete ureteral occlusion is an uncommon postprostatectomy disorder, with the exception of the inflammatory type of occlusion that may follow any type of prostatic operation. If intolerable colic, complete non-visualization by intravenous urography, or over-whelming kidney infection supervenes, relief by ureteral retrograde catheter intubation becomes mandatory. If catheterization fails, surgical relief is necessary. This type of secondary surgery depends upon individual circumstances, so generalizations on this topic are neither appropriate nor helpful.

13. Acute urinary retention following removal of the catheter

When the patient is unable to void voluntarily after 12 days of catheter drainage, a single dose of a *cholinergic drug* is given in combination with warm baths and ambulation. If these measures are futile, a urethral catheter of small caliber (No, 16 F) is reinserted and is left indwelling for at least 3 days. **Intermittent catheterization should** *not be employed*. It is exceedingly rare that a patient is unable to void following 3 additional days of catheter drainage. When this situation does develop, panendoscopy of the lower urinary tract is indicated. In rare instances, *a mechanically obstructing flap of tissue must be removed with a resectoscope.*

14. Surgical trauma of the rectum

The surgeon's fear and anticipation of urinary or fecal fistulae, or combinations of both, are **unwarranted**. This danger, like that of urinary incontinence, exists mainly in the *imagination of surgeons who seldom or never employ perineal techniques for prostatic surgery*. Precise surgical technique, prompt recognition of rectal injuries, and adequate surgical correction, combined with proper postoperative care, preclude persistent fistulae. The preferred techniques for perineal surgery depicted here are such that quick inspection of the ventral rectal wall will either give assurance that rectal injury has not occurred or will permit immediate recognition of an injury that must be repaired.

The postoperative care of the patient with a rectal injury repaired during perineal prostatic surgery is as follows :

♦ *Before the patient is removed from the operating table,* **the rectal sphincter should be dilated** with the hand to a diameter of approximately 10 cm. This can be accomplished by gradual and persistent dilatation over a period of 5 minutes. The procedure causes a certain degree of paralysis, which may last for several days.

♦ The patient should be started on a program of **bowel sterilization** medication at once. A **soft rectal tube** is inserted 15 cm and is left inlying.

♦ *Parenteral feeding* is prescribed for 2 or 3 days, followed by 1 week of a nonresidue liquid oral diet. The drain in the perineum is removed 1 week after surgery. The urethral catheter is left indwelling for 2 weeks and is removed only if there is no evidence of rectocutaneous fistula formation. The rectal tube is removed 1 week after surgery, and is changed whenever it becomes occluded. **The rectal tube is never irrigated.**

Radical Prostatectomy: the Pros and Cons of the Perineal versus Retropubic Approach

H.A. Frazier, J. E. Robertson and D. F. Paulson

From the Division of Urology, Department of Surgery and Cancer Center Database, Duke University Medical Center, Durham, North Carolina, USA

Within the current urological community the majority of urologists use the radical retropubic approach, which is due in part to the familiarity with the surgical anatomy as well as the development of the nerve sparing technique first described by Walsh et al.

The perineal approach fell out of favor due to the lack of familiarity with the perineum as well as the perception that patients had more difficulty with impotence and cancer control with this approach.

We have described various minor modifications to the perineal approach, which have allowed the surgeon to preserve the neurovascular bundle and achieve a tight vesicourethral anastomosis.

This study was performed to evaluate the short-term differences between the 2 operations. Since radical perineal prostatectomy and radical retropubic prostatectomy are performed at our institution, a direct comparison was possible between both surgical approaches.

MATERIALS AND METHODS

A retrospective review was performed on all clinical stage T_1 (A) or T_2 (B) prostate cancer cases that were treated at Duke University Medical Center during 1988 and 1989. A total of 173 patients was believed to have clinically organ confined prostate cancer (stage T_1 or T_2), and was subsequently treated with staging pelvic lymph node dissection and radical prostatectomy.

Of this patient population 122 were treated by radical **perineal** prostatectomy (**group 1**) by the senior author (D. F. P.) and 51 were treated by radical **retropubic** prostatectomy (**group 2**) by 1 of 3 senior staff surgeons.

Patient age ranged from 44 to 79 years (mean 65 years).

The **selection** of radical perineal versus radical retropubic prostatectomy was dependent upon the preference of the surgeon.

To provide equivalence, **operative time** and anesthesia time were determined only in those group 1 patients who underwent a staging lymphadenectomy and radical perineal prostatectomy, and includes time to reposition and drape. Operative time was from lymphadenectomy incision to perineal closure.

Each patient who was potent preoperatively was counseled as to the potential for unilateral preservation of the neurovascular bundle on the side opposite the sentinel lesion. Potency postoperatively was defined by the patient stating that adequate vaginal penetration had been achieved during the follow up period. Rigidity was not evaluated.

Each parameter was evaluated statistically and compared between the 2 groups.

Table 1. In-hospital complications

	N° Pts
Group 1 (4%):	
Epididymo-orchitis	1
Bacteremia	2
Abdominal incision abscess	1
Perineal incisional abscess	1
Group 2 (4%):	
Aspiration pneumonia,	
Myocardial infarction	1
Death secondary to cardiac arrest	1

Table 2. Long term complications

	Goup 1 N° (%)	Group 2 N° (%)
Stress incontinence	5 (4)	2 (4)
Anastomotic stricture	8 (7)	4 (8)
Bladder stones	0 (0)	1 (2)
Urethrorectal fistula	1 (1)	0 (0)
Total	14 (12)	7 (14)

RESULTS AND DISCUSSION

There was no difference in the median age and the stage of the tumor in the 2 groups. The pathological specimens were evaluated for invasion into the various surrounding structures as well as positive or negative surgical margins. There was no statistical difference between the 2 groups with regard to bladder or urethral involvement as well as invasion into the seminal vesicles or penetration through the capsule. Group 1 had a 29% incidence of positive margins while group 2 had a 31% incidence of positive margins (p = 0.803).

There was a 4% incidence of short-term complications in both groups (table 1).

The incidence of long-term complications was similar between both groups as well, with a 12% incidence in group 1 and 14% in group 2 (table 2).

The data in this study established a distinct difference in estimated **blood loss** and transfusion rate between groups 1 and 2. Patients in group 1 (perineal) had a median

estimated blood loss of 565 cc, while for those in group 2 (retropubic) it was 2,000 cc (p <0.001). This difference in estimated blood loss was supported by the difference in total number of units transfused while in the hospital. Group 1 patients required a median of 0 transfusions while in the hospital, while group 2 patients required a median of 3 units of blood (p <0.001). There was no difference between the 2 populations with regard to the preoperative hematocrit but there was a statistically significant difference in the postoperative and lowest in-hospital hematocrit in favor of group 1.

While the blood loss for the group 2 patients was approximately 85% greater than that reported by others, the figures of Walsh reflect the experience of a surgeon specifically skilled in radical retropubic prostatectomy just as our figures reflect those of a surgeon preferring radical perineal prostatectomy. The institutional experience reported reflects the statewide experience of North Carolina urologists. The demonstration of reduced blood loss and decreased transfusion requirements with radical perineal prostatectomy is important for a generation of surgeons unfamiliar with these specific advantages of this operation, and for a population of patients concerned about the risks of hepatitis and the acquired immunodeficiency syndrome associated with heterologous blood transfusions.

A common perception is that **operative and anesthesia time** would be extended in group 1 (perineal) due to the sequencing of staging pelvic lymph node dissection, repositioning and radical perineal prostatectomy. Operative and anesthesia times were remarkably similar for both groups.

Potency after radical prostatectomy has become a major issue in recent years. Of the patients in this population who underwent a nerve-sparing radical perineal prostatectomy (group 1) 77% are potent with adequate vaginal penetration more than 1 year postoperatively. Potency information was not routinely available on patients in group 2 and, therefore, a direct comparison is not possible. However, the postoperative potency rate in group 1 is comparable to the 72% figure previously published by Walsh. Thus, comparable potency rates are possible with the perineal approach.

The question arises: *is radical perineal prostatectomy an adequate cancer operation?* There was no difference in the incidence of invasion into the bladder, urethra or seminal vesicles, or penetration through the capsule of the prostate. *The incidence of positive surgical margins was nearly identical in the 2 patient populations*, with 29% in group 1 and 31% in group 2 (no statistically significant difference). These data would argue that radical perineal prostatectomy and radical retropubic prostatectomy are equivalent cancer operations for adenocarcinoma of the prostate. A recent review of the survival data for patients who had been treated with radical perineal prostatectomy at Duke revealed results comparable to other previously published studies using the radical retropubic approach. The short followup in this patient population does not allow adequate evaluation of survival differences between the 2 groups. To date, there is no difference in incidence of recurrence, progression or probability of survival.

In summary, radical perineal prostatectomy is an excellent operation for treatment of adenocarcinoma clinically confined to the prostate. The *perineal approach* offers *cancer control equivalent* to the retropubic approach with a *smaller transfusion requirement*. There is *no increased operative or anesthesia time* required in repositioning the patient from the supine position to exaggerated lithotomy. The radical retropubic and radical perineal prostatectomies have a *similar incidence* of short-term and long-term *complications*. There is *no difference in the histopathological cancer control*, progression or probability of survival. Radical perineal prostatectomy offers an excellent opportunity for cancer control.

DOCUMENTATION

PAULSON, D. F.: Radical perineal prostatectomy. Urol. Clin. N. Amer., 7: 847,1980.

PAULSON, D. F., MOUL, J. W. AND WALTHER, P. J.: Radical prostatectomy for clinical stage TI-2NOMO prostatic adenocarcinoma: long-term results. J. Urol., 144: 1180,1990.

RAINWATER, L. M. AND SEGURA, J. W.: Technical consideration in radical retropubic prostatectomy: blood loss after ligation of dorsal venous complex. J. Urol., 143:1163,1990.

NESS, P. M., BOURKE, D. AND WALSH, P. C.: A randomized trial of preoperative hemodilution vs. predeposit autologous transfusion in radical retropubic prostatectomy. J. Urol., part 2,145: 292A, abstract 319, 1991.

Staging Laparoscopic Pelvic Lymph Node Dissection: Comparison of Results with Open Pelvic Lymphadenectomy

Raul Para, Charles Andrus and John Boullier

Division of Urology, Department of Surgery, Saint Louis University Schoool of Medicine, Saint Louis, Missouri, USA

The accurate definition of pelvic lymph node status is of paramount importance before institution of any treatment is considered for prostate cancer.

Presently, no non invasive imaging modality has the level of accuracy to identify precisely disease in the lymph nodes. Computerized tomography, MRI or lymphangiography, with or without thin needle aspirates, all lack in sensitivity or specificity, firmly establishing surgical pelvic lymphadenectomy as the most precise method to assess the status of the lymph nodes. Nevertheless, **standard open pelvic lymphadenectomy** is not without **potential morbidity**, and **errors** in frozen sections diagnosis can occur as well.

Laparoscopic pelvic lymph node dissection has been suggested as a **less invasive substitute** to the seemingly more traumatic open standard dissection routinely performed.

Such technique seems **potentially attractive:**

1. for patients scheduled to undergo **radiation therapy**

2. for those considered to be at **high risk for nodal metastases** because of:

a. elevated acid phosphatase levels and normal bone scans.

b. marked elevation of serum PSA levels without other evidence of disease spread

c. poorly differentiated or high volume tumors in whom the more accurate pathological assessment of pelvic lymph nodes by means of permanent sections could prove beneficial, while sparing them the disadvantages of an open procedure.

We undertook this prospective study with the purpose of determining if the **laparoscopic approach** to the pelvic lymph node dissection was **as precise as the standard open lymphadenectomy.**

Group 1 consisted of 12 stage T1-2 patients who underwent a standard open modified lymph node dissection and,

Group 2 included 12 stage T1-2 patients who underwent laparocopic lymph node dissection.

Patients were **similar** in regard to age, clinical stage and grade, but the laparoscopic lymph node dissection patients had significantly higher levels of PSA, suggesting a more advanced disease in this group.

The location and size of the incisions for insertion of trocars is represented on Figure 1, and the limits of the dissection on Figure 2. In all patients in the laparoscopic group who subsequently underwent a radical prostatectomy, we explored carefully the area of the lymph node dissection for remaining lymphatic tissue.

In no instance was additional lymphatic tissue obtained by open dissection. **Operative time** for laparoscopic lymph node dissec-

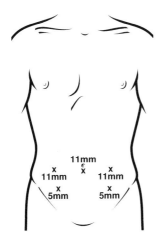

Figure 1. Location for insertion of trocars and corresponding diameters used.

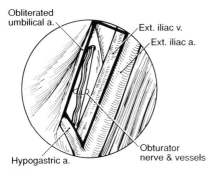

Figure 2. Diagrammatic representation of laparoscopic field of dissection. Margins of dissection are delineated by heavy line. a., artery, v., vein, Ext., external

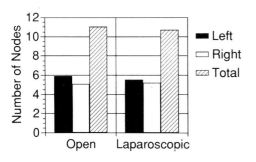

Figure 3. Overall total amount of nodes harvested and number retrieved by side of dissection and technique.

tion ranged from 80 to 315 minutes with an average time of 185 minutes. Patients who did not go on to have a radical prostatectomy because they had positive nodes were **discharged home** the morning after surgery and were able to resume their normal activites within 72 hours in the laparoscopic group, contrasting with a hospital stay of 4 days and a convalescence period of 2 weeks in the open lymph node dissection group.

Lymph node metastases were found in 1 patient in the open lymph node dissection group and in 3 patients in the laparoscopic lymph node dissection group, obviating the need for radical prostatectomy in these patients. As shown on fig. 3 the average **number of lymph nodes retrieved** in the two groups was similar. In no patient did the laparoscopic technique miss any positive lymph nodes.

The advent of laparoscopic lymph node dissection has opened the possibility of performing a surgical dissection **equal to the open method** but with the possible advantages of decreased patient morbidity, hospital stay and cost.

Its superiority is particularly evident in patients who will altogether be spared an open procedure by this technique:

• patients scheduled for radiation therapy in whom an assessment of the status of the lymph nodes is preferable, and

• the patients at high risk of lymph node positivity in whom the demonstration of invasion of the lymph nodes in this less invasive fashion will spare a radical prostatectomy.

What about Laser in the Treatment of Localised Prostate Cancer?

H.O. Beisland

Department of Urology, Aker Hospital, Oslo, Norway.

We have studied the feasibility and efficacy of a treatment modality combining a *radical TURP* and *laser coagulation of the prostatic fossa* with a neodymium-YAG laser (which produces a homogeneous coagulation of the 5-6 mm of tissue remaining after the TURP) in 118 patients.

The treatment procedure is carried out in *two separate steps.*

1. An experienced urologist performs *as radical a TURP as possible* : if preoperative transrectal ultrasound shows too much residual tissue, a second TURP is recommended.

2. Three to five weeks later, the *entire surface of the prostatic fossa is coagulated with a laser* power of 45-50 W in overlapping single pulses of 4 s. In order to properly treat the apex, we have found it necessary to systematically introduce a cystoscope by a small suprapubic cystotomy. Caution has to be exercised on the posterior fossa to avoid rectal injury.

Results compare satisfactorily with those of external beam or implant irradiation. Of *104 T1b-T2 (A2-B2) patients,* mean age 69 years, followed up 6-98 months, actuarial disease free survival rate is 98% at 1 year, 90% at 2 years, 89% at 3 years and 88% in the 4-8 year period. Twelve patients have failed, most at 12-24 months, 6 locally and 6 distally.

Complications have been few and the procedure, which lasts some *35-40 min*, is virtually devoid of complications: no bleeding, Foley catheter removed the morning after surgery, and the patient home the next day.

We had only one serious complication, a case of urinary incontinence, which required the implantation of an artificial sphincter.

In conclusion, combined TURP-and-YAG laser irradiation is a promising treatment option for localised prostate cancer, one which needs to be compared to other established treatment modalities in prospective trials.

DOCUMENTATION

BEISLAND H.O. : Neodymium-YAG laser in the treatment of localized prostatic cancer. Acta Urol Belgica 57, 709-713 (1989).

What can Cryosurgery Offer in the Treatment of Prostatic Cancer?

G. Rigondet , J.M. Salé, R. Claude, H. Roubertie et J.M. Cheveau.
Polyclinique St. François et Centre Anticancereux Joseph Belot, Montluçon, France

Cryosurgery has not received a lot of attention in the treatment of prostate cancer. Yet, its effects are potent, and well defined: central necrosis due to blood vessel thrombosis, surrounded by a peripheral zone with hyperhemia (which might potentiate radiotherapy and chemotherapy) (Figure 1).

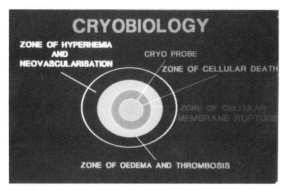

Figure 1. Cryobiology

It is mainly meant for high risk patients, as no anesthesia is needed. There is no post-operative bleeding, even in patients with clotting disorders.

1. Treatment with palliative intent:

a) effects on bladder outlet obstruction: comparable to those of TURP, without the inherent risk of the operation.

b) effects on cancer progression: considering that the main indication for the operation was poor performance status and severe and/or multiple associated illnesses, this study cannot safely assess the contribution of cryosurgery to cancer control.

Nevertheless, we have observed a serendipitous beneficial effect on bone pain in several patients, for which we cannot give a definite explanation, due to the anecdotal nature of these observations.

c) immunolgic effects: some authors have assumed an enhancement of the immune anticancer response in patients receiving cryosurgery. No indisputable proof, however, exists so far to that effect.

2. Treatment with intent to cure:

As a first line of treatment, we have offered patients who were a contraindication for radical prostatectomy an association of high voltage radiation therapy and cryosurgery, mostly in stage T2 patients, but also in a few T3.

With regard to cancer control, with a follow up limited to 4 years, we have 80% good results, as appreciated on the digital rectal examination and a significant drop in the PSA level (which occurs much faster than with radiation therapy alone).

With regard to voiding symptoms, urinary retention has resolved in 70% of the cases, with an overall rate of satisfactory results of 56%.

In this curative setting, we think cryosurgery has a role to play in a very select group of patients who are a contraindication to radical prostatectomy: prospective trials are needed to confirm these initial observations

DOCUMENTATION

LOENING S. et al. Perineal cryosurgery of prostate cancer. 1981, Urology 17, 12-14.

Palliative Surgery for Advanced Prostatic Cancer

J. Vicente, P. Laguna
Fundation Puigvert, Barcelona, Spain

I. INTRODUCTION

In patients with "terminal" prostatic cancer presenting with urethrovesical obstruction and in cases of hormone-resistant prostatic cancer with ureteric obstruction, anuria or oliguria, urologists are obliged to choose between letting the patient die and a more active, although palliative, therapeutic approach.

1. Urethrovesical obstruction is frequent: many patients (18 to 72%) develop obstruction at some time during the course of the disease. This obstruction presents either in the form of acute urinary retention (15% of cases in our experience), requiring emergency urethral catheterisation, or chronic retention. As the majority of these patients are already hormone-resistant, hormone therapy is of no benefit and radiotherapy induces major adverse effects (urethral stricture in 8% of cases, proctitis, etc.).

2. Ureteric obstruction occurs in 10 to 30% of cases of advanced prostatic cancer, presenting in the form of anuria or progressive hydronephrosis that may lead to renal failure.

II. PALLIATIVE SURGERY FOR VESICOURETERIC OBSTRUCTION

Transurethral resection of the bladder neck and prostatic urethra provides a rapid and effective solution to acute (33 cases) or chronic (219 cases) urinary tract obstruction. The details of the technique depend on the morphology and extent of the prostatic tumour.

1. When the morphological abnormality is confined to the bladder neck or posterior urethra, the resector can be mobilised relatively easily and the resection technique is similar to that used for benign prostatic hypertrophy (40% of our cases). This technique ensures wide resection of tumour tissue preventing further episodes of obstruction in patients with a long life expectancy (Figure 1).

2. When advanced prostatic cancer has extensively invaded the bladder neck and prostatic urethra (60% of our cases), the technique consists of cone resection : a large, funnel-shaped communication is made between the bladder and the healthy urethra. The resection starts in the upper quadrants, where the structures are better preserved, followed by clockwise resection with increasing depth, as far as the verumontanum. The major problems consist of the difficulties of mobilising the resector, inadequate evaluation of the tissue to be resected (by digital rectal examination) and the lack of precise limits due to invasion of the verumontanum (Figure 1)

3. In conclusion : transurethral resection is an excellent method to relieve bladder neck obstruction. In our experience, it was successful in 83% of cases and patency was maintained for an average of 21 months. The survival was 44% with a mean follow-up of three years. This is a minimally invasive technique responsible for an immediate postoperative mortality of only 0.8%. However, transurethral resection for advanced prostatic cancer is a controversial technique for the following three reasons :

a) **Dissemination of metastases,** raised by several authors, but rejected by others. In our series of 113 patients with stage T3 cancer, operated by transurethral resection, only 43 cases (38%) developed metastases over a mean observation period of 33 months. In view of the late onset of metastases, the absence of any statistically significant difference between patients in whom prostatic cancer is diagnosed by TUR or by needle biopsy and even the preselection of patients reported in certain series, the pejorative role of TUR in relation to dissemination of cancer cells appears to be dubious.

b) **Need for repeated TURs :** in our experience, the resection had to be repeated in 33% of cases after an average of three years. The need to repeat the procedure depends on the aggressiveness of the initial transurethral resection and the subsequent course of the disease. We therefore recommend that as much tissue as possible be resected during the first operation.

c) **Complications of TUR** : severe bleeding was observed in 4.5% of our cases and 8.6% of patients developed postoperative urinary incontinence. However, the incidence of incontinence after radiotherapy is 8% and is often accompanied by local disturbances : proctitis, radiation cystitis, etc.

In our experience, transurethral bladder neck resection has a low mortality and morbidity and can be repeated several times, although a small number of patients with a very poor general status will not support such surgery. ***Two alternatives are available*** in these patients :

◆ *Insertion of an intraprostatic stent*, performed under local anaesthesia and even on an outpatient basis. The technique is simple, based on conventional instruments. We have performed this technique in 7 cases : the stent was kept in place with comfortable micturition for an average of 8.2 months in five patients and in two patients, the prosthesis had to be removed due to intolerance.

◆ ***Prostatic hyperthermia.*** Due to the poor blood supply of the prostatic cancer, hyperthermia induces histological changes of cell damage. However, clinical studies have failed to demonstrate any changes in DNA or any significant variations in PSA. Out of 7 patients with an indwelling catheter, only two regained spontaneous micturition.

III. PALLIATIVE SURGERY FOR URETERIC OBSTRUCTION

Involvement of the upper urinary tract by advanced prostatic cancer may present in the form of *anuria* (11 cases), a real urological emergency, or in the form of *progressive dilatation* leading to oliguria and chronic renal failure (35 cases). The aetiological mechanism is generally compression of the intramural segment of the ureter. Deep transurethral resection of the trigone is a helpful procedure to help restoring ureteral patency as it make stenting possible.

1. Anuria requires urinary diversion by nephrostomy and, whenever possible, antegrade introduction of a double J stent . This manoeuvre was only possible in two of our 11 cases as ureteric catheterisation was impossible because of deformation of the tri-

Palliative surgery in prostatic cancer

1. Transurethral surgery of prostate cancer

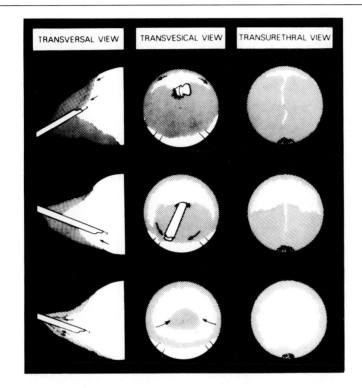

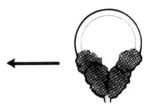

1. When the morphological abnormality is confined to the bladder neck or posterior urethra, the resector can be mobilised relatively easily and the resection technique is similar to that used for benign prostatic hypertrophy (40% of our cases).

2. When advanced prostatic cancer has extensively invaded the bladder neck and prostatic urethra (60% of our cases), the technique consists of cone resection .

2. Endoscopic surgery of ureteric obstruction

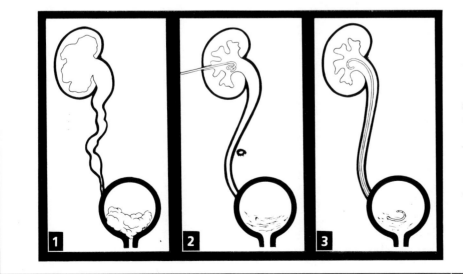

In anuria or Obstructive oliguria, We are active supporters of trigone resection with restoration of ureteric patency preceded by nephrostomy and followed by insertion of a double J stent

gone. Consequently, these cases were treated by deep resection of the trigone and antegrade or retrograde insertion of an internal diversion double J stent (Figure 2).

This technique ensured stable urinary tract patency, although five patients died during the first two months. The remaining patients had a mean survival of 8 months, while 22% were still alive with their disease at five years.

2. Obstructive hydronephrosis due to hormone-resistant prostatic cancer must not be considered to be a terminal situation, although the prognosis depends on the invasive nature of the tumour. We are active supporters of trigone resection with restoration of ureteric patency preceded by nephrostomy and followed by insertion of a double J stent (Figure 2).

This technique was followed by correction or stabilisation of the serum creatinine in 26 of the 35 cases treated. The ureter remained patent for an average of eighteen months and the mean survival was 22 months. The patients obtained a good quality of life without having to be admitted to hospital.

DOCUMENTATION

BANUS J.M., PALOU J., CORTADELLAS L., MOROTE J.Y., SOLER ROSELLO A. Transurethral resection of the ureteral meatus invaded by carcinoma of the prostate : a new approach. Eur. Urol. 13 : 344, 1987.

ELYADERANI M.K., GABRIELE O.F., KANDYARI S.J. y BELIS J.A. Percutaneous nephrostomy and antegrade ureteral stent insertion. Urology 20 : 650, 1982.

KYNASTON H.G., KEEM C.W., MATTHEWS P.N. Radiotherapy for palliation of locally advanced prostatic carcinoma. Br. J. Urol. 66 : 515, 1990.

SCHMID H.P. The problem of obstruction in prostate cancer. Urological Research 19 : 323, 1991.

STABLES D.P. Percutaneous nephrostomy : techniques, indications and results. Urol. Clin. North. Am. 9 : 15, 1982.

VICENTE J., CHECHILE, G., VALENZUELA R. Résultats du cathéter en double J comme dérivation urinaire interne. J. Urol. Nephrol. 93 : 553, 1987.

II

RADIOTHERAPY

Radiation Technique

M. A. Bagshaw, G.R. Ray, R. S. Cox

Department of Radiation Oncology, Stanford University School of Medecine,
Stanford, California, USA

The basic technique includes: tumor localization, treatment planning, and therapy.

1. Tumor localization

Several techniques for tumor localization have been employed over the years. These included **orthogonal radiography** with the patient in the treatment position, **using contrast media** in the rectum, bladder, and urethra for precise delineation of anatomy, supplemented by **CT scanning** and, more recently, **magnetic resonance imaging**.

2. Radiation therapy routines

Two general radiation therapy routines have been utilized.

Linear accelerators with photon energies of approximately 4 Mv at 80 cm SAD, and 5 and 6 Mv at 100 SAD have been used exclusively.

a) Radiotherapy of prostatic region

The original routine which was applied in over 300 patients included irradiation to the prostate and the prostatic region only, with either a 360° rotational or a bilateral (left and right) moving beam arc technique.

In that technique, 7600 rad was delivered to the prostatic region in 7 1/2 weeks at the rate of 200-225 rad per day calculated to a volume of tissue of 6 to 8 cm in diameter.

b) Radiotherapy of lymph nodes

In more recent years, first and occasionally second echelon lymph nodes have been included in the treatment plan, necessitating a 4-fieldbox technique to treat the first echelon lymph nodes of the pelvis as well as the prostate. In some instances the treatment has extended to include the para-aortic lymph nodes as well. When the adenopathy is treated, the box technique is utilized first to approximately 2600 rad, at which point a coned down booster dose is delivered to the prostate only for 2000 rad, using left and right 120° moving arc therapy, and then the treatment program is expanded to the original 4-fieldbox to include the entire pelvic first echelon lymphatic drainage system (Figure 1). This program delivers 7000 rad in 7 weeks to the prostate and 5000 rad in 7 weeks to the first echelon adenopathy. When the para-aortic lymph nodes are also included, 5000 rad are delivered to the para-aortics.

This program has been extremely well tolerated, with only a rare instance of prolonged urinary discomfort or morbidity, usually associated with pre-therapeutic transurethral resection. More explicit technical detail has been published previously (Bagshaw, 1980, 1984, 1985).

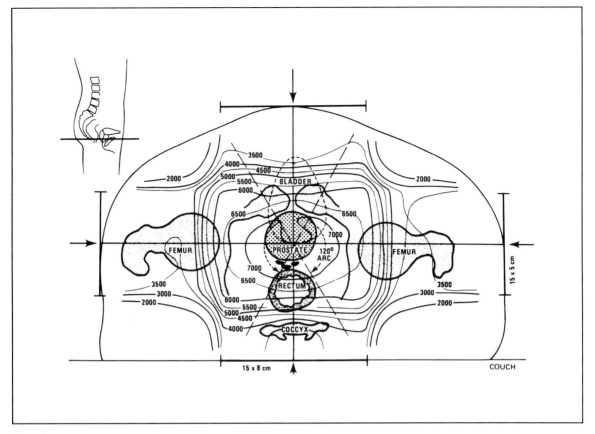

Figure 2. Composite isodose curve for treatment of carcinoma of the prostate taken at the level of the prostate. The first 2600 rad are delivered by the AP-PA and right and left lateral fields comprising the 4-field pelvic box technique. The next 2000 rad are delivered with fields of reduced cross-section using left and right 120° moving beam arcs. The final 2400 are delivered by the original 4-field box technique yielding 5000 rad in 7 weeks to the pelvic nodes and 7000 rad in 7 weeks to the prostate.

Radiation Sequelae

M. A. Bagshaw, G.R. Ray, R. S. Cox

Department of Radiation Oncology, Stanford University School of Medecine,
Stanford, California, USA

Adverse sequelae in the Stanford series were reported in 1976.

In that review based on 430 patients (Stage T1, T2, and T3-T4 inclusive), **urethral stricture** was encountered in 16 or 3.7%. The incidence of stricture was related to multiple pre-radiotherapeutic transurethral resections of the prostate.

In a study by Pilepich, post irradiation urethral stricture was noted in 5.2% and proctitis in 4.5% of the patients.

One patient with persistent tumor required a colostomy, and three had fecal stress incontinence and also urinary stress incontinence.

In the Patterns of Care outcome studies drawn from 163 randomly chosen radiation therapy facilities, **major complications** following radiation therapy which required hospital admission occurred in 28 of 619 (4.5%) of the stage T2, and T3-T4 patients evaluated. These involved urinary tract in 13, the bowel in 8, and both in 3. Sixteen required surgical intervention and one was fatal.

It appears that the **risk of incontinence** is significantly less following radiotherapy than following prostatectomy. This is certainly true in the Stanford series. Bowel complications appear somewhat greater after irradiation; however, with current radiation techniques, these are rare and can usually be attributed to persistent tumor.

A recent Stanford survey, summarized in Table 1, will be the subject of a later comprehensive report. This survey confirmed our clinical impression that adverse sequelae are less frequent and less severe than was the case more than 10 years ago. There does not appear to be a stage or grade shift in the patient profile and, therefore, **this reduction in sequelae is attributed to improvement in radiation technique.**

Table 1 does not include a cohort of 91 protocol patients treated during this same time period because they had all received a **transperitoneal lymph node staging** procedure, and in some the radiation dose to the para-aortic nodes was carried to 5500 rad. A substantially higher incidence of small bowel damage requiring surgical correction occurred in this selected cohort. Transperitoneal staging with extensive node dissection was abandoned in favor of retroperitoneal limited node sampling in appropriate cases, i.e., only a minority of non-protocol patients had any staging procedure, and the para-aortic radiation dose was reduced to 5000 rad in 5 weeks. In these cases "persistent" refers to symptoms of greater than 2-year duration, and "transient/severe" refers to symptoms requiring hospitalization and surgical correction. The most common symptom was some manifestation of urinary obstruction requiring transurethral resection. In this analysis, no at-

Table 1. Radiation sequelae -Prostatic cancer (non protocol patients)

1/65 – 12/74: 431 patients	Intestinal	Urological	Other (edema)
Persistent	22/431 5.1 %	33/431 7.7 %	7/431 1.6 %
Transient severe	6/431 1.4 %	14/431 3.2 %	1/431 0.2 %
1/75 – 12/84: 289 patients			
Persistent	7/289 2.4 %	14/289 4.8 %	4/289 1.4 %
Transient severe	0	7/289 2.4 %	1/289 0.3 %

Chi Square = 9.08; Two-tailed P-value = 0.0026

tempt was made to distinguish between symptoms caused by tumor and those caused by the treatment. Often the distinction is impossible in patients with large destructive neoplasms. It is of interest that a statistically significant reduction in sequelae has occurred in the most recent decade.

Preservation of erectile potency is possible in a substantial number of patients after x-irradiation. Previously, we have reported preservation of potency in about 60% of the candidates. In a more recent survey, we noted preservation of potency at 15 months post-radiation treatment in 86% of 430 patients, most of whom claimed potency prior to radiation. Within this group were a few patients who had a chief complaint of impotence and in whom erectile potency returned after irradiation. Fifty per cent of the patients maintained erectile potency for at least 7 years, and slightly more than 30% maintained potency for the duration of their survival beyond 7 years.

Changes in technique at Stanford which have greatly improved patient tolerance and presumably reduced later serious sequelae include :

1) No more than **200 rad per day** tumor dose;

2) **Precision linear accelerator field design** employing individualized molded cerrobend collimators with exclusion of the posterior wall of the rectum in the lateral radiation fields;

3) **Treatment of all fields every day** (5 days per week, Monday through Friday),

4) Introduction of the **booster dose** to the prostate at mid-course of treatment;

5) **No more than 7000 rad in 7 weeks to the restricted prostatic region**, and **5000 rad in 5 weeks to the remainder of the pelvis;**

6) **Protection of testes** in a special lead shield.

DOCUMENTATION

ALLAIN YM, BOLLA M, DOUCHEZ J, et al: Cancer de la prostate: Résultats de la radiothérapie: Étude inter-centres. Bull Cancer Paris 72:559, 1985.

BAGSHAW MA: Current conflicts in the management of prostatic cancer. Int J Radiat Oncol Biol Physics, 12:1721,1986.

BAGSHAW MA: External beam irradiation of prostatic cancer. In Coffey DS, Resnick MI, Dorr FA, et al (eds): A Multidisciplinary Analysis of Controversies in the Management of Prostate Cancer. New York, Plenum Publishing, 1988, p 85.

BAGSHAW MA, Cox RS, Ray GR: Status of radiation treatment of prostate cancer at Stanford University. NCI Monographs 7: 47, 1988.

Complications of

Radiation Therapy :

William U. Shipley
J of Urol 147,929, 1992

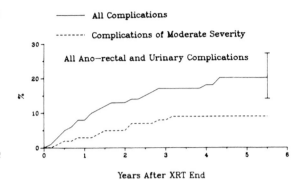

Figure 1. Actuarial incidence of complication as function of time after irradiation (XRT).

Radiation oncologists, like urologists, have made major improvements in treatment administrations during the last decade leading to a reduction in morbidity from radical surgery and radical radiotherapy. Figure 1 from the M.D. Anderson Hospital series documents a cumulative risk of all complications as being 18% up to 5 years when the curves reach a plateau and a cumulative incidence of 7% of complications of moderate severety: 2% are anal/rectal complications and 5% are urinary complications. This graph represents data from prospective analysis of 289 patients with followup on all patients who were treated for a 5-year period at that institution beginning January 1, 1984.

This level of complications is consistent with that reported recently by the Radiation Therapy Oncology Group (RTOG) in 1,020 irradiated patients evaluated prospectively on RTOG protocols from 1976 through 1983 with a minimum followup in surviving paitents of 7 years. A 3.3% incidence of intestinal complications of moderate severity or worse and a 7.7% incidence of urinary complications of moderate severity or worse were reported. The RTOG patients had a 1.1% incidence of severe complications requiring major surgical intervention or prolonged hospitalization. In a further analysis of the RTOG population base of a subset of 193 patients who died of prostate cancer a moderate or major urinary or intestinal complication following radiation therapy developed in 21 (11%) (Figure 2.)

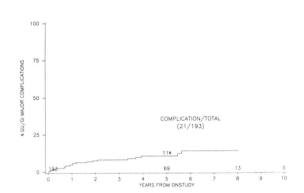

Figure 2. Actuarial incidence of moderate or major complications as function of time following radiation therapy in subset of 193 patients subsequently dying of prostate cancer either as primary or secondary cause in series reported by Lawton et al (personal communication from Dr. James Cox, Chairman, Radiation Therapy Oncology Group). GU/GI, genitourinary/ gastrointestinal.

Interstitial Irradiation Using I-125 Seeds

W. F. Whitmore, Jr., B. Hilaris, P. Sogani, H. Herr, M. Batata, W. Fair.
Urologic Service, Memorial Sloan Kettering Cancer Center, New York, USA

Interstitial implantation of I-125 seeds in the treatment of selected patients with prostatic cancer has been under investigation at Memorial Sloan-Kettering Cancer Center (MSKCC) since 1970. .

I. MATERIALS AND METHODS

This is an analysis of survival and recurrence experience with the first 164 patients treated in the interval 1970 through 1975, all of whom have been **followed for a minimum of 10 years.** This cohort of patients includes 99 patients with stage T2 disease and 65 with stage T3 -4 disease.

1. Case selection

Case selection varied during the period of this study. In general, the selected **patients had stage T2 or small T3 lesions** and an estimated life expectancy greater than five years. Local tumor categorization (Figure 1) was determined by digital rectal examination in conjunction with cystoendoscopy under anesthesia.

Patients with **T1 lesions were excluded** since the usual prior transurethral prostatic resection (TURP) was judged or assumed to have left insufficient residual prostate for satisfactory implantation.

Larger stage T3 tumors were usually judged unsuitable for implantation if there was palpable extension laterally into the levator muscle, apically outside the prostate, or extensively into the seminal vesicles. The subjectivity of local tumor categorization by digital rectal palpation is an acknowledged limitation of this study.

2. Technique

Radioactive iodine implantation is performed **through a retropubic approach immediately following bilateral pelvic lymph node dissection.** Low energy I-125 seeds are implanted in a rigidly defined pattern. Multiple implant needles are placed into the prostate at regular intervals. A **finger in the rectum** is important to guide the needle so that the seeds are not placed adjacent to the rectal wall.

A specially designed instrument is employed to deposit 40 to 70 seeds in vertical rows at regular intervals as the needle is withdrawn. The **dosage of irradiation must be homogeneous to avoid "cold spots"** within the neoplasm. Currently, 18,000 rad to the periphery of the tumor over a 1-year period is considered optimal. This is **equivalent** in its biologic effects on tissue to a dosage of approximately **8,000 rad external beam irradiation** at standard fractionations.

II. RESULTS

1. Progression rate

Figures 1 and 2 relate progression to **tumor stage and lymph node status** , respectively. Examined independently, each variable apparently **influences the progression** rate in a logically predictable fashion. A Cox regression analysis of these variables in the first 100 of these patients has indicated the **dominant role of lymph node status** in future progression. The **ominous implications of lymph node metastasis are highlighted in the subset of patients with T2a-b (B1-B2), grade I or II tumors** (Figure 2).

At 10 years 34% of 24 T2a lesions and 74% of 52 T2b lesions have progressed (Figure 1). When patients with positive nodes are excluded, **the progression rate for the combined T2a and T2b N0 categories at 10 years is 46%** (Figure 2).

2. Survival

Figures 3 and 4 relate overall survival to **tumour stage** and regional **lymph node status,** respectively. Survival may have been favorably influenced by endocrine therapy, usually utilized only for symptomatic metastases or more rarely for local progression with or without metastasis.

Survival for T2 a-b lesions or for T2c and T3 lesions shows remarkable overall similarity, respectively (Figure 3), the implication being that endocrine therapy may have obliterated any survival differences projected from the respective progression rates (Figure 1).

Figure 4 demonstrates the **adverse impact of lymph node metastasis on survival in the selected subset of patients with grade I or II T2 lesions.**

3. Status at 10 years of 164 patients

Table 1 provides an analysis of the status relative to prostatic cancer in the 164 patients at 10 years. Only 5 of 64 T3 category patients were alive and apparently well at 10 years but these 5 were among the 26 N0 patients. Local recurrences (with or without metastasis) were evident in 5 of 24 T2a lesions and in 61 of the 140 T2b, T2c and T3 lesions.

III. DISCUSSION

Other pertinent analyses remain to be carried out on this group of patients. Nevertheless, several observations may be offered from the data presented:

a) Tumour category and lymph node status, analyzed independently, influence prognosis following I-125 implantation. Based on a previous analysis of some of these patients, **lymph node status is the major determinant of prognosis.**

b) Patients with **grade I or 2 T2a-b** lesions without recognized lymph node metastases **achieved 54% 10 year apparent disease free survival** although prostatic biopsies were not done.

c) **Incidence of local failures in patients with T2c or T3 lesions is disappointing.**

d) Although lymph node metastasis clearly indicates a poor prognosis after I-125 implantation, a significant number of patients **without recognized lymph node metastases develop evidence of disease progression.** To what extent **recognized or unrecognized locally presistent (or "recurrent") tumour contributes to distant failures remains uncertain.**

e) The **downward slope of all of the progression and survival curves,** at least up to 10 years, is evident and emphasizes **the necessity for a longer follow up** to evaluate fully whatever impact the treatment

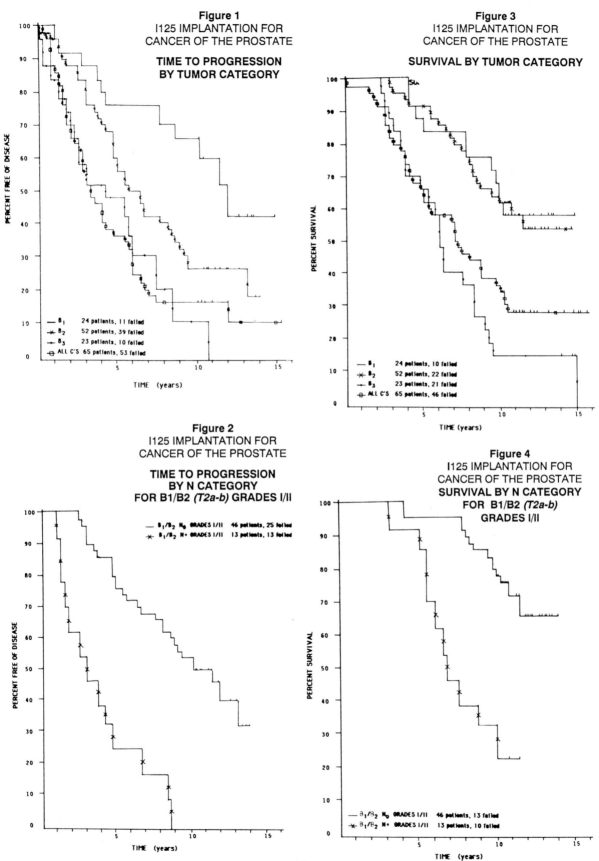

Figure 1
I125 IMPLANTATION FOR
CANCER OF THE PROSTATE

TIME TO PROGRESSION
BY TUMOR CATEGORY

- B₁ 24 patients, 11 failed
- B₂ 52 patients, 39 failed
- B₃ 23 patients, 10 failed
- ALL C'S 65 patients, 53 failed

Figure 3
I125 IMPLANTATION FOR
CANCER OF THE PROSTATE

SURVIVAL BY TUMOR CATEGORY

- B₁ 24 patients, 10 failed
- B₂ 52 patients, 22 failed
- B₃ 23 patients, 21 failed
- ALL C'S 65 patients, 46 failed

Figure 2
I125 IMPLANTATION FOR
CANCER OF THE PROSTATE

TIME TO PROGRESSION
BY N CATEGORY
FOR B1/B2 (T2a-b) GRADES I/II

- B₁/B₂ N₀ GRADES I/II 46 patients, 25 failed
- B₁/B₂ N+ GRADES I/II 13 patients, 13 failed

Figure 4
I125 IMPLANTATION FOR
CANCER OF THE PROSTATE
SURVIVAL BY N CATEGORY
FOR B1/B2 (T2a-b)
GRADES I/II

- B₁/B₂ N₀ GRADES I/II 46 patients, 13 failed
- B₁/B₂ N+ GRADES I/II 13 patients, 10 failed

61

Table 1. Status at 10 years of 164 patients

Category	NED	LRO	DMO	B	U	Total
T2a (B1) N0	13	3	3	2	1	22
T2a (B1) N+	0	0	2	0	0	2
T2b (B2) N0	12	9	6	8	2	37
T2b (B2) N+	0	1	9	4	1	15
T2c (B3) N0	2	3	5	2	0	12
T2c (B3) N+	1	1	5	4	0	11
T3 (C) N0	5	5	7	7	2	26
T3 (C) N+	0	5	15	12	7	39

may be having on the course of the disease.

The lack of routine prostatic biopsies, the criteria employed to define local and distant progression, the failure to utilize elevations of the serum acid phosphatase as a criterion for inoperability or disease progression, the confounding effect of endocrine therapy on survival, the absence of 15 years follow up data are amongst a number of shortcomings in the present analysis.

What seems unequivocal is that *some patients with apparently localized prostatic cancer survive without evidence of disease progression for at least 10 years after this method of treatment.* To what extent this fortunate state is a consequence of the treatment and to what extent a function of the natural history of the cancer is uncertain.

DOCUMENTATION

WHITMORE WF Jr: 1980 Interstitial radiation therapy for carcinoma of the prostate. The Prostate 1:157-168.

GROSSMAN HB, BATATA MA, HILARIS BS and WHITMORE WF Jr: 1982 I-125 implantation for carcinoma of the prostate. Further follow-up of first 100 cases. Urology 20:591-598.

HILARIS BS, WHITMORE WF, CHU FCH, MOSTOFI FK, KAZAM E, YEH SDJ, MORSE M, YAGODA A, HALL EJ, ANDERSON LL, BATATA MA, HERR HW, SOGANI PC, NISAR SYED AM, NORI D, ROTMAN M, VIKRAM B, ALFIERI A: 1983 Brachytherapy Oncology-1983 Edited by Basil S. Hilaris and Mostafa A Batata. Published by Memorial Sloan-Kettering Cancer Center,NY,NY.

Combined Interstitial and External Irradiation for Prostatic cancer

C. E. Carlton, Jr., P. T. Scardino

Department of Urology, Baylor College of Medicine, Houston, Texas.

I. INTRODUCTION

There is very good evidence to support the concept that irradiation therapy can destroy prostatic cancer. Patients with localized disease can be cured with radiotherapy.

Since 1965, at our institution, we have treated most patients who have localized prostatic cancer with *a combined approach* utilizing *implantation of radioactive gold seeds* into the prostate *followed by external beam irradiation*.

II. RATIONALE

By combining gold seed implantation with external beam irradiation, we proposed to deliver a *definitive* dose of irradiation to the prostate with *fewer complications* than with external beam irradiation alone. A dose of approximately 3000 rad was delivered by direct retropubic implantation of solid Au-198 seeds, and an additional 4000 to 5000 rad were given with external irradiation (Figure 1).

Virtually all the radiation from Au-198 has dissipated by 14 to 21 days, so that accurate radiation injury can be detected in time to adjust the planned course of external irradiation so that the side effects are minimized.

Because the half value layer (or effective depth of penetration of the radiation from Au-198 grains) is relatively long and because of the high energy of the grains used and the large field of radiation around each, the gold implant requires only a few (six to 10) grains and can be completed in a few minutes. Precise placement of the grains is not so critical, bleeding and operating time are minimal, and exposure of personnel to radiation is brief.

The combined treatment offers the advantage of accurate surgical staging, precise treatment to the palpable tumor mass, and flexible adjustment of the timing and dose of external therapy to the tolerance and needs of each patient. The radiopaque seeds offer an aiming point for external therapy, assuring treatment to the full extent of the tumor with minimal complications.

III. INDICATIONS

1. Candidates have clinical stage T1b, T2a-c and T3a

Definitive radiotherapy does not seem appropriate for stage T1a tumors, since the malignant potential of this tumor is quite low. Stage T3b-c tumors (> 6 cm) are too bulky for cure but may be palliated with radiotherapy. Candidates for definitive radiotherapy should have clinical stages T1b, T2a-c and T3a tumors, without clinical evidence of metastases. They should have a life expectancy of at least 5 years and have

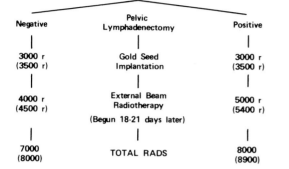

Figure 1. Treatment protocols used at Baylor College of Medicine for the combined therapy of localized prostatic cacer. Figures in parentheses indicate increased dose employed since 1980

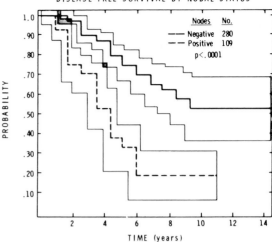

Figure 2. Disease-free survival by nodal status. Patients with positive nodes fare significantly worse than patients with negative nodes. Nodal status was the most powerful prognostic factor in this group of patients.

Table 1. Determinate survival rates by stage and for the overall group of 501 patients

Clinical Stage	DETERMINATE SURVIVAL Observed survival rate					
	5 years		10 years		15 years	
	N	%	N	%	N	%
T1b	101	89.1 ± 6.2	29	75.9 ± 15.9	1	0
T2a	19	100.0	9	100.0	3	66.6 ± 54.4
T2b	111	92.8 ± 3.0	28	67.9 ± 17.6	4	50.0 ± 50.0
T2c	72	88.9 ± 7.4	19	73.7 ± 20.2	2	0
T3a	94	78.7 ± 8.4	23	34.8 ± 19.8	4	0
Overall	397	88.2 ± 3.2	106	66.1 ± 9.2	14	28.6 ± 24.2

Table 2. Actuarial survival rate for overall goup at 5 and 10 years

OVERALL ACTUARIAL SURVIVAL		
	N	%
5 years	324	99 ± 3
10 years	117	61 ± 7

Table 4. Disease-free survival as calculated by life table analysis

OVERALL ACTUARIAL N.E.D. SURVIVAL		
	N	%
5 years	233	76 ± 5
10 years	31	46 ± 8

Table 3. Disease-free survival as calculated by the determinate methods.

Clinical stage	DETERMINATE SURVIVAL Observed disease-free survival			
	5 years		10 years	
	N	%	N	%
T1b	81	69.1 ± 10.0	21	38.1 ± 21.2
T2a	16	75.0 ± 21.6	6	66.6 ± 35.4
T2b	100	66.6 ± 9.3	21	33.3 ± 20.6
T2c	65	56.9 ± 12.2	16	12.5 ± 16.5
T3a	90	36.7 ± 10.2	23	17.4 ± 15.8
Overall	352	58.2 ± 5.3	87	28.7 ± 9.7

had no prior pelvic irradiation or significant rectal or bladder disorders which could be exacerbated by the irradiation.

2. A transurethral resection should be performed if retention is imminent

Patients who present in urinary retention or with severe obstructive voiding symptoms must be managed cautiously, since *no technique of radiotherapy is advisable while the patient has an indwelling urethral catheter.* If the patient cannot void, or if retention is imminent, a transurethral resection of the prostate (TURP) should be performed.

Endocrine therapy is sometimes successful in relieving or preventing obstruction and can be stopped when the radiotherapy is complete.

If a TURP is necessary before radiotherapy, the prostatic urethra should be allowed to re-epithelialize completely, *over a 6-week period, before therapy is begun* to minimize the irritative voiding symptoms so often associated with radiotherapy and to **decrease** *the risk of bladder neck contracture.*

3. Management of pelvic lymph nodes.
Management of the pelvic lymph nodes remains controversial. Some argue that once the tumor metastasizes to the pelvic nodes, the disease is systemic and incurable; therefore, pelvic nodal irradiation is futile.

However, Paulson et al. (1982) have demonstrated in a controlled trial of patients with *proven positive pelvic nodes*, that full pelvic and para-aortic irradiation *results in a longer tumor-free interval compared to no treatment.* In addition, our own data, as well as that of others, have shown long-term disease-free survival in approximately 15% to 20% of patients with positive nodes. Consequently, there is reason to argue that pelvic nodal metastases alone do not preclude cure and that these nodes should be

treated by irradiation or node dissection or both, along with the primary tumor.

IV. TECHNIQUE

1. Gold seed implantation

Gold seed implantation is performed through a retropubic aproach. Following a *limited staging pelvic lymph node dissection,* 6 to 10 radioactive gold seeds are implanted, aiming for a total of 3500 rad (Figure 1). A simple implant needle is used.

Although the seeds are placed throughout the gland, an effort is made to cluster the seeds in the area of the palpable tumor.

2. Adjuvant external beam radiotherapy

Beginning *14 to 21 days after the implant*, when radiation from gold grains is exhausted, a course of external beam radiotherapy is given using the 7 MeV linear accelerator.

Treatment protocol is summarized by Figure 1.

V. COMPLICATIONS

Complications of gold seed implantation and external beam irradiation have been few and are quite comparable to those reported for I-125 implantation. Three deaths were reported in our series (523 patients).

VI. RESULTS

We have recently reviewed the results of combined gold seed and external irradiation in 523 patients.

a) Survival

The actuarial and determinate overall survivals are depicted in Tables 1 and 2. There is very little difference in survival as calculated by these two methods.

b) Disease-free survival

Disease-free survival for clinical stage T1b was poor, with 35% developing recurrent tumor within 5 years (Tables 3 and 4). Those with stage T3 tumors demonstrated progressive treatment failure over the period of follow-up, 40% being free of disease at 5 years and 3% at 10 years. However, patients with the well defined *1.5-cm nodule of prostatic cancer fared well,* with 81% free of disease at 5 years and 50 % at 10 years, a rate comparable to the expected survival for the age-matched general population of males aged 63 in 1975.

c) Survival by nodal status.

Although survival correlated with stage and grade, the greatest impact on survival was the presence and extent of lymph nodal metastases.

1. If the *nodes were negative*, 53 ± 9% survived for 10 years free of disease.

2. if the *nodes were positive,* only 18 ± 6% were free of disease at 10 years (Figure 2).

3. Patients with a **single positive node** (N1) had a significantly (p < 0.01) **better disease-free survival rate** than those with more than one node (N2-4).

Hence, some patients with minimal nodal metastases do achieve long-term survival free of tumor with no other systemic therapy. *Nodal metastasis, in our experience, is not synonymous with systemic disease*. But whether such long-term "cures" can be attributed to the natural history of the disease, the lymphadenectomy, or the pelvic radiotherapy remains unclear.

VII. SUMMARY

Definitive radiotherapy, administered by a variety of modalities, can control localized prostatic cancer in the majority of patients when adequate dosages are used. Success often depends upon the biologic potential of the tumor as much as the specifics of the treatment techniques. *Survival free of recurrent or residual tumor* is best when the tumor is palpable and confined to the gland (stage T2), and worse for stage T1b and T3, for high grade tumors, and for those with positive nodes. *Complications* are relatively infrequent, although perhaps more common with definitive external beam irradiation alone. Erectile impotence occurs in 10% to 40%, but incontinence is very rare.

Surgical staging with pelvic lymphadenectomy is a crucial determinant of prognosis, allows adjustment of treatment portals and may offer some therapeutic benefit in those with minimal nodal involvement (N1).

DOCUMENTATION

CARLTON CE, Jr. Radioactive isotope implantation for cancer of the prostate? In Crawford ED and Borden TA (eds): "Genitourinary Cancer Surgery", Borden, Lea and Febiger, Philadelphia, 1982.

ELDER JS, JEWETT HJ and WALSH PC. Radical perineal prostatectomy for clinical stage B2 carcinoma of the prostate. J Urol 127:704-706, 1982.

GUERRIERO WG, CARLTON CE, Jr, and HUDGINS PT Combined interstitial and external radiotherapy in the definitive management of carcinoma of the prostate. Cancer 45:1922-1928, 1980.

JACOBI GH and HOHENFELLNER R. Staging, management and post-treatment re-evaluation of prostate cancer : Dogma questioned. In : Prostate Cancer, edited by G.H. Jacobi and R. HOHENFELLNER R, pp. 45-46, 212-214. Williams and Wilkins, Baltimore, 1982.

PAULSON DE et al. Extended field radiation versus delayed hormonal therapy in node positive prostatic adenocarcinoma. J Urol 127:935-937, 1982.

PAULSON DF et al. Radical surgery versus radiotherapy for adenocarcinoma of the prostate. J Urol 182:502-504, 1982.

SCARDINO PT, GUERRIERO WG and CARLTON CE, Jr. Surgical staging and combined therapy with radioactive gold grain implantation and external irradiation. In : Genitourinary Tumors Fundamental Principles and Surgical Techniques, edited by DE Johnson and MA Boileau, pp. 75-80. Grune and Stratton, New York, 1982.

Prognostic Value of Biopsy after Irradiation

U. E. Studer

Inselspital, Urologische Universitätsklinik, Bern, Switzerland

Before we can judge the prognostic value of post-irradiation biopsy, we first have to know:

1. From what point on should the biopsy be negative: immediately after irradiation treatment has been completed or later?

Cox et al. in 1977, in keeping with other published reports, demonstrated that the incidence of positive biopsy decreases with time. Directly after irradiation therapy, all prostatic biopsies are positive. After 12 to 18 months, half of them are negative. No further decrease can be observed beyond 2 years : *biopsies that are still positive after 2 years will continue to be positive.*

2. In which patients, or tumors, do post-irradiation biopsies become negative and in which ones do they remain positive?

Freiha and Bagshaw like other authors, demonstrated on the basis of their patients in Stanford, California, that the probability of a biopsy remaining positive increases in relation to tumor stage (Table 1). The more advanced the tumor stage, the more probable that the prostatic biopsy will not be negative. This produces a dilemma, as we know that patients with advanced tumor stages are the very ones that should be able to benefit from irradiation, since they are the ones that will most likely die from prostatic cancer.

3. Why does the rate of response to irradiation decrease with increasing tumor stage?

One possible explanation is that the tumor volume increases in higher stages. Pilepich et al. in 1987 investigated this correlation and found that local tumor control is relatively successful as long as the tumors are small, but begins to fail significantly as the tumor volume increases. Patients with large tumor volumes, in other words, those who should profit most from irradiation, are the ones with the highest rate of recurrence or persistence of cancer.

4. Does the reason for failure lie more in the dependence on tumor stage or on tumor volume?

The answer to this question is probably "neither nor", since in most cases both are ultimately the result of *the degree of differentiation*. This is corroborated by the work of Perez et al., who studied patients with

Table 1. Results of biopsy according to the stage of the primary tumor.

Stage	n	positive biopsy
T1b	1	0 (0%)
T2a	2	0 (0%)
Small T2b	8	3 (38%)
Large T2b	22	13 (59%)
T3	31	23 (74%)
Total	64	39 (61%)

the same local tumor stage and hence with comparable tumor volumes, but with different gradings. A comparison of well, moderately, and poorly differentiated carcinomas shows that the poorly differentiated tumors are clearly the ones that persist or recur locally. Accordingly, the further course of these tumors is also unfavorable. This observation applies for both stage T2 (B) and stage T3-T4 (C) tumors. The probability of being able to achieve local tumor control with irradiation is lowest for the poorly differentiated stage T3-T4 (C) tumor, i.e. the tumor with the worst prognosis. Also, there is a high probability that positive biopsies will be found in follow-up of these patients. Again, those patients with the worst prognosis are the ones in whom irradiation has the least chance of getting the tumor under control.

From this we can derive the following definition of patients *at risk of having persistent positive biopsies* after irradiation: patients with *advanced stages* of prostatic carcinoma or *larger tumor* volumes, such tumors *usually being poorly differentiated*.

5. Might age also play a role ?

Pilepich et al. [6] investigated the effect of irradiation in men over 70 and under 60 years of age and found no significant differences between the two groups with regard to local recurrence.

6. What is the significance of negative or positive post-irradiation biopsy?

If the biopsy is negative, the probability of recurrence is low. *If the biopsy is positive, the chance of local tumor relapse increases significantly with time*. A positive biopsy obtained 18 months after irradiation means that sooner or later we can expect to find local recurrence.

7. What are the consequences for the patients? Does this affect survival?

Leach et al., for instance, believed that pa-

tients with positive biopsies and those with negative biopsies ultimately would have the same chances of survival. Their findings, however, were based on only 40 patients. Extreme caution must therefore be exercised in interpreting such results, particularly when they do not (cannot) demonstrate any difference. It therefore comes as no surprise that Kuban et al. obtained very different results among their 295 patients who underwent external beam high-voltage irradiation for prostatic carcinoma : the 5-year survival of patients who had no local recurrence was 89%; in contrast, the probability of survival of those patients who had a positive prostatic biopsy after irradiation was only 66% (p < 0.001) after 5 years. This was comparable with the survival rates of those patients who suffered distant metastases after irradiation. Whether or not distant metastases existed at the time of positive biopsy is of secondary importance. These results clearly show that *a positive biopsy after external beam or interstitial irradiation ultimately means a poor prognosis* - as poor as it would be if the disease had already disseminated.

SUMMARY

Patients with prostatic carcinomas having a poor prognosis, that is, tumors that are initially advanced and/or undifferentiated, are more likely to suffer tumor persistence or local tumor recurrence after external beam (and/or interstitial) irradiation. The poor degree of differentiation is the main factor contributing to the unfavorable prognosis. A positive biopsy 18 months after irradiation means a poor prognosis, which is comparable with that of patients with confirmed metastases. In the latter patients *with local tumor persistence, the disease has usually already disseminated, even if no metastases are detected at the time of the positive prostatic biopsy*. Metastatic disease, however, should not be considered the failure of irradiation alone, *for at least in some cases distant micrometastases must have existed at the time of the local therapy.*

DOCUMENTATION

COX JD, STOFFEL TJ. The significance of needle biopsy after irradiation for stage C adenocarcinoma of the prostate. Cancer 40:156-169, 1977.

FREIHA FS, BAGSHAW MA. Carcinoma of the prostate: results of post-irradiation biopsy. Prostate 5:19-25, 1984.

KUBAN DA, EL-MAHDI AM, SCHELLHAMMER PF. Prognosis in patients with local recurrence after definitive irradiation for prostatic carcinoma. Cancer 63:2421-2425, 1989.

LEACH GE, COOPER JF, KAGAN AR et al. Radiotherapy for prostatic carcinoma: postirradiation prostatic biopsy and recurrence patterns with long-term follow-up. J Urol 128:505-508, 1982.

PEREZ CA, PILEPICH MV, ZIVNUSKA F. Tumor control in definitive irradiation of localized carcinoma of the prostate. Int J Radiat Oncol Biol Phys 12:523-531, 1986.

PILEPICH MV, BAGSHAW MA. Asbell SO et al. Definitive radiotherapy in resectable (stage A2 and B) carcinoma of the prostate. Results of a nationwide overall view. Int J Radiat Oncol Biol Phys 13:659-663, 1987.

ROBEY EL, SCHELLHAMMER PF. Local failure after definitive therapy for prostatic cancer. J Urol 137:613-619, 1987.

III

HORMONE THERAPY

Hormonal Physiology of the Prostate

S. Khoury, K Griffiths

Hôpital de la Pitié, Paris, France
Tenovus Institute, Cardiff, U.K.

I. PROSTATE AND TESTOSTERONE

The development and function of the prostate principally depend on circulating *testosterone*

a) *Castration before puberty* prevents the prostate from developing and reaching its functional maturity;

b) *Castration once the gland has reached maximum size* induces atrophy of the gland and arrest of secretory activity ;

c) *Administration of exogenous testosterone* to a castrated animal or man restores prostatic growth and secretory activity.

II. SYNTHESIS AND DISTRIBUTION OF ANDROGENS IN THE BODY

1. Origin of androgens

Circulating *androgens* can originate in either the testis or adrenal glands: 92 to 95% of androgens are secreted by the testes, while 3 to 7% originate in the adrenals (Figure 1).

The *testis* principally secretes testosterone and androstenedione. Very small quantities of DHT are secreted directly by the testis.

The *adrenals* principally secrete androstenedione (Δ4), dehydroepiandrosterone (DHEA) and DHEA sulphate. These androgens are synthesised from a common precursor : *cholesterol*. They are transformed into testosterone in target cells (adipose cells, prostate...) or peripherally (adipose cells).

2. Influence of the pituitary

Testicular androgens. Testosterone is secreted by the Leydig cells of the testis in response to a pituitary hormone, luteinizing hormone (LH). LH secretion is in turn controlled by LHRH (Luteinising Hormone Releasing Hormone) a neurohormone produced in the hypothalamus which reaches target cells in the anterior pituitary via the hypophyseal portal vascular system.

Adrenal androgens are secreted in response to ACTH, which is also controlled by a hypothalamic secretory factor (CRF) transported via the same pathway.

3. Role of prolactin

Prolactin, a pituitary hormone, affects the prostate in two ways (Figure 3) :

a) *indirectly*, by promoting the formation of androgens by the testes and adrenals ;

b) *directly*, by potentiating the action of testosterone on prostatic tissue, as prolactin promotes the uptake of testosterone by epithelial cells.

However, prolactin appears to play only an accessory role in the development of prostatic disease (benign prostatic hypertrophy or cancer).

Prolactin inhibitors have been used in the treatment of benign prostatic hypertrophy and prostatic cancer, but with limited results.

III. ACTION OF TESTOSTERONE

1. Circulating testosterone

98% of plasma testosterone and DHT are bound to a plasma protein.

◆ 57% of plasma testosterone is specifically and avidly bound to a specific protein present in the plasma called the Sex Hormone-Binding Globulin (SHBG). The SHBG level is increased by oestrogens.

◆ 40% is less specifically and less avidly bound to albumin and

◆ 1% is bound to corticosteroid binding globulin (CBG).

Only the **free fraction (2%)** (not bound to protein), is physiologically active, as only the free form is able to cross the cell membrane.

2. Testosterone acts via its active metabolite, dihydrotestosterone (DHT) (Figure 4).

Testosterone can only act at the cellular level after being transformed into DHT by an enzyme, *5α–reductase*. This transformation takes place on the nuclear membrane of target cells.

a) DHT is the principal hormone isolated from cell nuclei following the administration of testosterone.

b) There is a correlation between the degree of androgenic activity of steroids and their capacity to be transformed into DHT in the cells.

c) Subjects with congenital *5α–reductase* deficiency suffer from prostatic agenesis.

3. DHT selectively binds to a specific nuclear androgen receptor [AR] to form the DHT-AR complex.

Binding to AR conditions DHT action.

The activated AR can then bind to specific regions of the gene.

The interaction of the DHT-AR complex with the DNA in the nucleus influences gene expression. This elicits the synthesis of specific proteins corresponding to the specific function of the cell.

By a mechanism which is still poorly understood, this [DHT-receptor] complex induces transcription of messenger RNA which, on the ribosomes, codes for the formation of specific proteins responsible for the specific cellular response to hormonal stimulation.

4. Physiological variation in androgen levels

The plasma testosterone levels remain in the vicinity of 500 ± 270 ng/100 ml between the ages of 20 and 60 years. After this age, the levels start to gradually fall. This fall is accompanied by an increase in oestradiol levels. The *oestradiol/testosterone* ratio tends to increase at about the age of 60 years.

5. Metabolism of androgens

Circulating androgens are metabolised in the liver into 17-ketosteroids conjugated to glucuronic acid, while sulphoconjugates are derived from the adrenals. 30% of urinary 17-ketosteroids are of testicular origin, while 70% are of adrenal origin. In practice, it is impossible to distinguish between testicular and adrenal 17-ketosteroids, which is why 17-ketosteroid assay is an unreliable indicator of androgenic activity in man.

IV. ROLE OF OESTROGENS

Small amounts of oestrogen are present in men (100 ng/litre). They are principally derived from the peripheral *aromatisation* of testosterone in adipose tissues and from secretion by the testis.

Although oestrogens increase SHBG and decrease free circulating testosterone, endogenous oestrogens appear to play *a synergistic role to the action of androgens* on the prostate. The mechanism of this synergy is poorly understood, but appears to be due to an enhancing of the production of androgen-induced cell growth regulators mainly in the prostatic stroma, and possibly by increasing levels of androgen receptors.

The prostate is primarily androgen-dependent

It is well established by an accumulation of evidence from both human and animal studies that the growth, development, maintenance and function of the prostate gland are primarily dependent upon the concentration of plasma testosterone

Pre-natal development of the prostate is androgen dependent

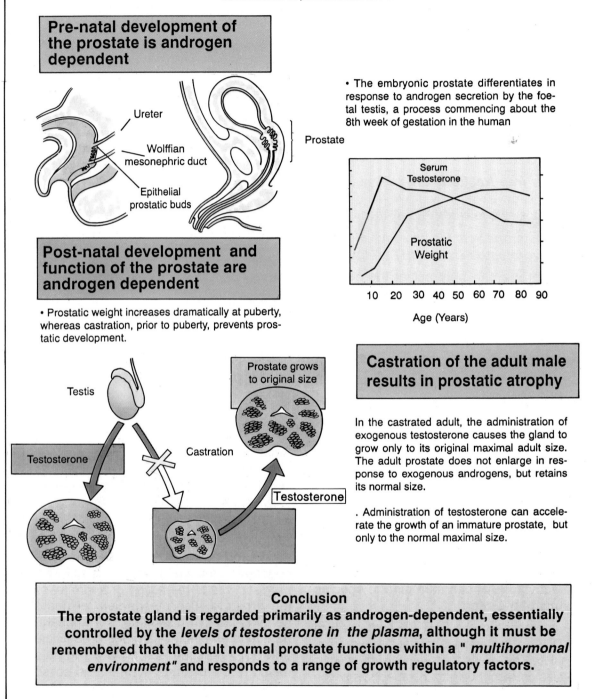

Ureter

Wolffian mesonephric duct

Epithelial prostatic buds

Prostate

• The embryonic prostate differentiates in response to androgen secretion by the foetal testis, a process commencing about the 8th week of gestation in the human

Serum Testosterone

Prostatic Weight

10   20   30   40   50   60   70   80   90

Age (Years)

Post-natal development and function of the prostate are androgen dependent

• Prostatic weight increases dramatically at puberty, whereas castration, prior to puberty, prevents prostatic development.

Testis

Testosterone

Castration

Prostate grows to original size

Testosterone

Castration of the adult male results in prostatic atrophy

In the castrated adult, the administration of exogenous testosterone causes the gland to grow only to its original maximal adult size. The adult prostate does not enlarge in response to exogenous androgens, but retains its normal size.

. Administration of testosterone can accelerate the growth of an immature prostate, but only to the normal maximal size.

Conclusion
The prostate gland is regarded primarily as androgen-dependent, essentially controlled by the *levels of testosterone in the plasma*, although it must be remembered that the adult normal prostate functions within a " *multihormonal environment"* and responds to a range of growth regulatory factors.

Origin of plasma testosterone

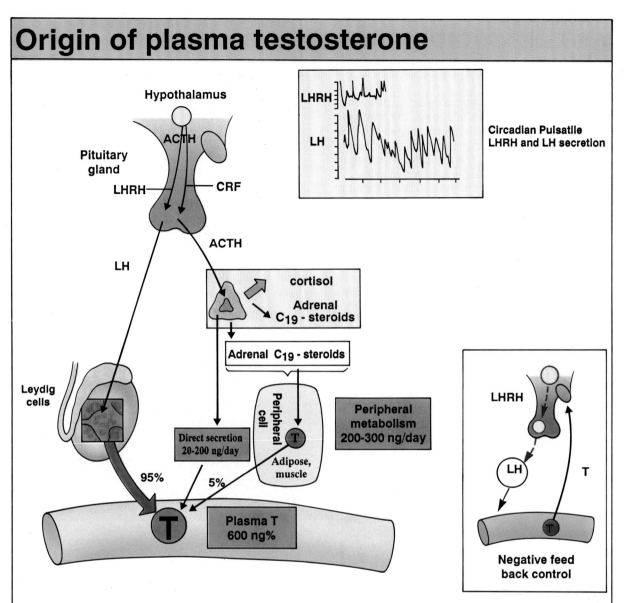

Hypothalamus

ACTH

Pituitary gland

LHRH — **CRF**

ACTH

LH

Leydig cells

cortisol

Adrenal C$_{19}$ - steroids

Adrenal C$_{19}$ - steroids

Peripheral cell

Peripheral metabolism 200-300 ng/day

Direct secretion 20-200 ng/day

Adipose, muscle

95%

5%

T

Plasma T 600 ng%

LHRH

LH

T

Circadian Pulsatile LHRH and LH secretion

LHRH

LH

Negative feed back control

The principal circulating androgen is testosterone (T). Circulating T is derived from two main sources :

❶ Testis.

The **testis** produces approximatively 95 % of the circulating testosterone (T). T is synthesised within the testis by the **Leydig cells.** The Leydig cells are stimulated by **gonadotrophins** (primarily luteinising hormone **LH**) to synthesise testosterone. The spermatic vein concentration of testosterone is 40 to 50 mg / 100 ml and is approximately 75 times higher than the level detected in the peripheral venous serum. LH secretion by the pituitary is under the control of a decapeptide released by the hypothalamus referred to as **LHRH** (Luteinising Hormone Releasing Hormone). LHRH is released in a **pulsatile manner** to promote a similar pulsatile production of LH. Androgens (and oestrogens) exert a **negative feed-back control** to regulate gonadotrophin secretion.

❷ Adrenals

Approximatively 5% of the circulating T originates from peripheral transformation (mainly in the adipose tissue) of adrenal C$_{19}$-steroids into testosterone. The secretion of C$_{19}$-steroids by the adrenal is under the control of ACTH.
The effects of a normal level of adrenal androgens on the prostate are not significant because adrenalectomy has very little effect on prostate size. Adrenals cannot prevent prostatic atrophy following castration.

Intraprostatic metabolism of testosterone

The free plasma T is the biologically active form. Of the total testosterone in plasma, 2% is free and it is this free fraction which is considered to be the biologically active moeity that passively diffuses into the prostate cells. The remaining testosterone is bound to to a specific protein present in the plasma called the Sex Hormone-Binding Globulin (SHBG) (57%), and to albumin (40%).

In prostatic cells T is metabolised into DHT, the active intracellular androgen by specific enzyme 5α-reductase

Testosterone is metabolised, within the prostate cells, to 5α-dihydrotestosterone (DHT), which has a greater affinity than testosterone for the intracellular androgen receptor protein. This conversion is mediated by an enzyme, 5α-reductase [5α-R] associated with the nuclear membrane. It is well accepted that DHT is the most active intracellular androgenic hormone.

DHT selectively binds to a nuclear specific Androgen receptor [AR] to form the DHT-AR complex.

The activated AR can then bind to specific regions of the gene.

The interaction of the DHT-AR complex with the DNA in the nucleus influences gene expression. This elicits the synthesis of specific proteins corresponding to the specific functions of the cell.

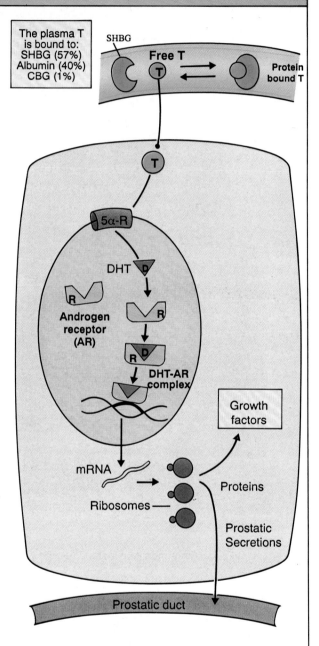

The plasma T is bound to:
SHBG (57%)
Albumin (40%)
CBG (1%)

The interaction of the DHT-AR complex with its specific gene (s) on the nuclear DNA molecule influences each of the genes to generate "messages" to produce a specific biological response corresponding to the gene function.

This is achieved by inducing the transcription of the gene into mRNA (messenger ribonucleic acid molecule) which is transported out of the nucleus, to the ribosome (the final site of protein synthesis) where the "message" is finally translated into a protein. The nature of this protein depends on the structure of the activated gene:

◆ **Secretory genes** will lead to the formation of a **secretory protein** which will be excreted by the cell.

◆ **Proliferation genes** will lead to the formation of a series of **growth factors** necessary for cell division and the homeostasis of the prostate.

Hormonal Treatment Rationale and Specific Hormone Therapy

S. Khoury

Urology Department, Hôpital de la Pitié, Paris, France

I. RATIONALE

1. Prostate cancer responds to "*androgen ablation*"

The landmark observations of Huggins and Hodges in 1941 regarding the efficacy of androgen-ablative or suppressive therapy in the treatment of metastatic prostate cancer established "androgen deprivation" as the mainstay of treatment for advanced prostatic carcinoma. Indeed, about 70% of patients so treated will exhibit beneficial responses of an objective and subjective nature, including:

1. a decrease in the size of primary and metastatic tumours;

2. reduction in the levels of serum prostatic acid phosphatase (PAP) and prostate-specific antigen (PSA);

3. decrease in bladder outlet and ureteric obstruction;

4. a partial reversal of myeloplasic anaemia;

5. relief of bone pain;

6. an improvement in appetite along with a general sense of well-being.

This approach was based on the logical hypothesis that prostate cancer cells retained some of the characteristics of nontransformed prostatic epithelium and would therefore undergo atrophy after androgen deprivation.

The duration of this response ranges from a few months to **several years,** with the majority of patients succumbing to the uncontrolled growth of **androgen-independent** disease (stage D3) within 6 to 18 months.

2. Hormonal escape

a. Prostate cancer cells are biologically heterogeneous (Plate 1)

As stated previously, about 30% of men with advanced-stage prostate cancer will not respond to androgen deprivation. Moreover, virtually all of the initial responders (if they survive long enough) will eventually demonstrate disease progression. The initial absence of response, and the secondary hormonal escape strongly suggest that prostate cancers are biologically heterogeneous, consisting of **androgen-dependent** (androgen-responsive), and **androgen-independent** (androgen-unresponsive) cell populations. Androgen-deprivation therapy destroys androgen-dependent cells, but has no direct influence on those that are androgen-independent which continue to grow and are responsible for disease progression.

b. What is the mechanism of emergence of such heterogeneity ?

Several hypotheses have been proposed to explain the development of hormone-insensitive cells. The most likely hypothesis, the **clonal selection model**, assumes that

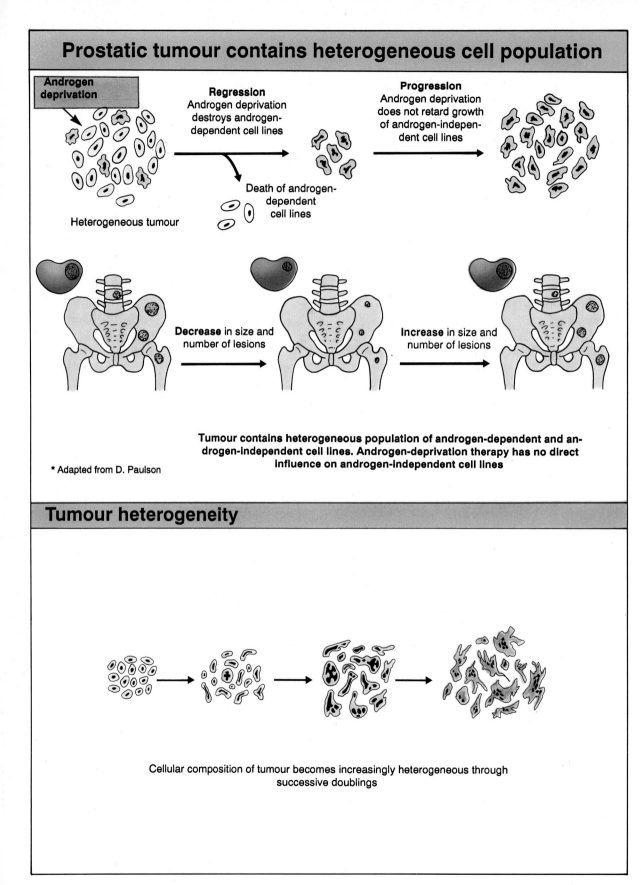

Prostatic tumour contains heterogeneous cell population

Androgen deprivation

Heterogeneous tumour

Regression
Androgen deprivation destroys androgen-dependent cell lines

Death of androgen-dependent cell lines

Progression
Androgen deprivation does not retard growth of androgen-independent cell lines

Decrease in size and number of lesions

Increase in size and number of lesions

Tumour contains heterogeneous population of androgen-dependent and androgen-independent cell lines. Androgen-deprivation therapy has no direct influence on androgen-independent cell lines

* Adapted from D. Paulson

Tumour heterogeneity

Cellular composition of tumour becomes increasingly heterogeneous through successive doublings

Specific hormone therapy

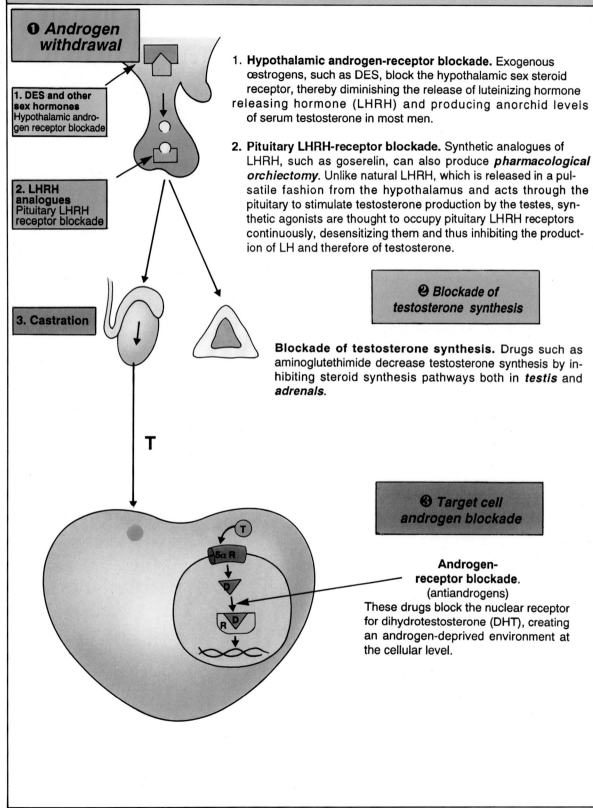

❶ Androgen withdrawal

1. DES and other sex hormones
Hypothalamic androgen receptor blockade

2. LHRH analogues
Pituitary LHRH receptor blockade

3. Castration

1. **Hypothalamic androgen-receptor blockade.** Exogenous œstrogens, such as DES, block the hypothalamic sex steroid receptor, thereby diminishing the release of luteinizing hormone releasing hormone (LHRH) and producing anorchid levels of serum testosterone in most men.

2. **Pituitary LHRH-receptor blockade.** Synthetic analogues of LHRH, such as goserelin, can also produce *pharmacological orchiectomy*. Unlike natural LHRH, which is released in a pulsatile fashion from the hypothalamus and acts through the pituitary to stimulate testosterone production by the testes, synthetic agonists are thought to occupy pituitary LHRH receptors continuously, desensitizing them and thus inhibiting the production of LH and therefore of testosterone.

❷ Blockade of testosterone synthesis

Blockade of testosterone synthesis. Drugs such as aminoglutethimide decrease testosterone synthesis by inhibiting steroid synthesis pathways both in *testis* and *adrenals*.

T

❸ Target cell androgen blockade

Androgen-receptor blockade. (antiandrogens)
These drugs block the nuclear receptor for dihydrotestosterone (DHT), creating an androgen-deprived environment at the cellular level.

prostate cancers become heterogeneous soon after malignant transformation, with the emergence of hormone-independent cell lines. This is due to the genomic disturbances that arise because of the genetic instability, changes that are characteristic of most tumour systems.

3. Dedifferentiation of the cell population and loss of hormone dependence increases with tumour growth.

Longstanding clinical observations show that as *tumour volume* increases with sucessive doublings, the likelihood of progression to higher-stage hormone insensitive disease also increases.

A number of studies have demonstrated that the frequency of *aneuploidy* is higher with advancing stage of human prostate cancer. Available evidence also suggests that the presence of highly aneuploid cell populations (triploid or hexaploid) is associated with more aggressive tumour systems manifesting relative hormone insensitivity.

II. SPECIFIC HORMONAL TREATMENT

Hormonal treatment used in clinical practice aims either to *ablate* the androgens in the host, or to *block their action* on the androgen receptors in the tumour. Plate 2 presents a classification based on their primary mechanism of action. Table 1 summarises the current procedures for first line endocrine treatment. These will be discussed in more detail in the following chapters.

Table 1. Current first line endocrine treatment

Androgen withdrawal

    Bilateral orchidectomy

    LHRH agonists

    Oestrogens

Androgen blockade: Antiandrogens

    Steroid : Cyproterone acetate

    Pure : Flutamide, Nilutamide

Combination treatment

    Castration (surgical/medical) and antiandrogens

DOCUMENTATION

DENIS L. Current strategies in hormonal manipulation of advanced prostate cancer. Current Opinion in Urology 1991, 1:16-20.

MCCONNEL J.D. Physiologic basis of endocrine therapy for prostate cancer , Urol Clinic North Am 1991, 18, N°1, 1-14.

Oestrogens in the Treatment of Prostatic Cancer

K. Griffiths, S. Khoury

Tenovus Institute, Cardiff, U.K.
Hôpital de la Pitié, Paris, France

I. MECHANISM OF ACTION

Although the principal mechanism of action of diethylstilboestrol (DES) appears to be exercised indirectly by decreasing testicular testosterone secretion, by pituitary suppression of LH secretion, evidence also exists for a direct action of DES on both prostate and testis. Moreover, DES increases the circulating levels of SHBG thereby indirectly decreasing the plasma free testosterone fraction.

At high doses, DES can decrease DNA synthesis (Plate 1).

II. DES AND PROSTATIC CANCER

1. Clinical results

DES was the most widely used reference oestrogen for the treatment of prostatic cancer. This synthetic oestrogen is the least expensive and the most effective of the oestrogens used. DES, at the dose of 3 mg/day appears to be effective, less so at 1mg/day. A dose of 5 mg, or the administration of very high doses (> 100 mg) does not appear to be any more effective than 3 mg/day.

The Veterans Administration studies (VACURG) provided a most instructive contribution to our understanding of endocrine treatment in prostatic cancer.

a) First VACURG study

The first study, which commenced in 1960, was directed to patients with *stage A and B* cancer randomised to receive either radical prostatectomy with placebo, or radical prostatectomy with 5 mg of DES per day.

Patients with **stage C and D** disease were randomised to receive placebo, 5 mg of DES per day, castration with placebo or castration with 5 mg of DES per day.

The results of this first study showed that the overall survival was less favourable in stage A patients who received 5 mg of DES, but no significant difference was observed in stage B patients.

The survival was also less favourable in stage C patients who received castration together with 5 mg of DES, in comparison with those who received placebo alone, or castration with placebo.

No significant differences were observed amongst the various treatment schedules for stage D patients.

The study of the survival curves, taking into account causes of death, showed that stage C and D patients who received 5 mg of DES, in comparison with the placebo group, had a significantly higher mortality from cardiovascular complications (most of the deaths occurred during the first year) and a lower death rate from prostatic cancer.

These results were most surprising. At the time, oestrogens were thought to have a favourable effect on cardiovascular disease as reflected in the fact that randomised clinical studies were then being conducted to evaluate oestrogen treatment as a means of preventing the progression of cardiovascular disease (Coronary Drug Project Research Group 1970).

Oestrogens Mechanism of action

1. Principal central action

The principal mechanism of action of oestrogens is central: they block LHRH secretion by the hypothalamus, which results in inhibition of LH secretion by the pituitary and testosterone secretion by the testis.

They also have a **peripheral action:**

❶ they increase TeBG, thereby decreasing the plasma free T,

❷ they have a direct action on the testis by decreasing T secretion

❸ they have a direct antiandrogenic action on the prostate.

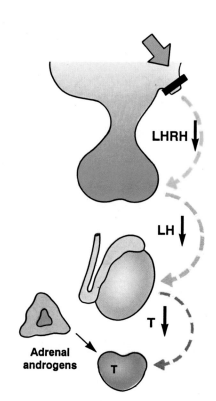

LHRH ↓

LH ↓

T ↓

Adrenal androgens

T

High doses

↓

DNA synthesis
(used in hormone-resistant cases)

2. Accessory peripheral action
Peripheral action of oestrogens

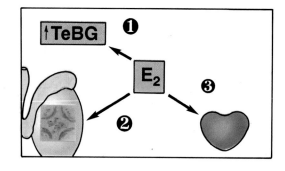

↑TeBG ❶

E₂

❸

❷

**Hormonal consequences
of oestrogen therapy**

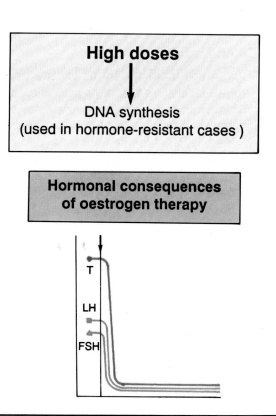

T

LH

FSH

Table1. Deaths by stage, treatment, and cause in VACURG Prostate Study 1

	Stage 1		Stage 2				Stage 3				Stage 4	
	Px+P	Px+E	Px+P	Px+E	P	E	O+P	O+E	P	E	O+P	O+E
Number of patients	60	60	85	94	262	265	266	257	223	211	203	216
Cause of death												
Cancer of the prostate	3	2	8	2	46	18	35	25	105	82	97	82
Cardiovascular causes	20	25	25	32	88	112	95	108	55	76	56	59
Other	7	10	9	12	43	50	54	48	29	23	29	40
Total deaths	30	37	42	46	177	180	184	181	189	181	182	181

Table 2. Deaths by stage, treatment, and cause in VACURG Prostate Study 2

	Stage 3. DES				Stage 4. DES			
	Placebo	0,2 mg/day	1,0 mg/day	5,0 mg/day	Placebo	0,2 mg/day	1,0 mg/day	5,0 mg/day
Number of patients	76	73	73	73	53	52	55	54
Cause of death								
Cancer of the prostate	11	9	3	3	21	28	17	14
Cardiovascular causes	15	14	18	31	10	7	10	10
Other	11	19	14	7	9	1	4	7
Total deaths	37	42	35	41	10	36	31	31

The first VACURG study revealed another surprise : the overall survival of the patients treated with placebo was equivalent to that of the patients receiving endocrine therapy. In reality, this conclusion was biased, as most of the patients with Stage C cancer (70%), and all of the patients with stage D cancer initially treated with placebo *subsequently received endocrine therapy* when disease progression made this treatment necessary. The definitive results were still tabulated however in the form of initial randomisation, i.e. placebo. For this reason, the VACURG results did not show that placebo was equivalent to endocrine therapy in terms of overall survival but that *deferred endocrine therapy was as effective as early endocrine therapy* initiated at the time of diagnosis.

b) Second VACURG study

The second VACURG study commenced in 1967 and was designed to demonstrate :

a) That in patients with stage A and B cancer, radical prostatectomy could offer an advantage in terms of survival over placebo alone.

b) That low doses of DES were more effective than doses of 5 mg, to control progression of prostatic cancer without inducing cardiovascular complications.

Patients with stage C and D disease were randomised to receive either placebo, 0.2 mg, 1 mg, or 5 mg DES per day. In patients with stage C and D disease, the dose of 1 mg of DES was as effective as the dose of 5 mg and significantly more effective than the 0.2 mg dose, or placebo, in the prevention of death from prostatic cancer without being associated with an increased frequency of cardiovascular mortality.

c) Third VACURG study

A third study commenced by VACURG in 1969, compared the efficacy of oestrogens other than DES, or of certain progestins, administered orally, with that of 1 mg of DES per day.

Patients were randomised to receive either 1 mg of DES per day, 30 mg of medroxyprogesterone acetate per day, 1.25 mg of premarin for one month, followed by 2.5 mg per day and 30 mg of medroxyprogesterone acetate with 1 mg of DES per day.

The results did not reveal any significant advantage in terms of overall survival, or cancer death, for these therapeutic protocols when compared with 1 mg of DES per day.

III. DISCUSSION

Although the VACURG studies profoundly influenced our ideas about endocrine therapy in prostatic cancer, they nevertheless gave rise to certain invalid interpretations of the results.

1. Hormonal treatment and survival

The first invalid interpretation related to the statement that **endocrine therapy did not prolong patient survival.** This is not true. As revealed by the first study, all patients with stage D cancer initially randomised to receive placebo subsequently received endocrine therapy. Consequently, this study was unable to conclude that placebo was as effective as endocrine therapy in terms of overall survival, but that **deferred endocrine therapy was as effective as early endocrine therapy.**

The second VACURG study also showed that endocrine therapy prolonged survival of patients with Stage D cancer. In contrast with the first VACURG study and bearing in mind that oestrogens could be dangerous, all of the patients with stage D disease in this second study, placed on placebo and who continued to progress, were not systematically placed on oestrogens and some of them continued with placebo treatment. Consequently, the 2nd study showed that 19% of patients placed on placebo were alive compared with 44% and 45% of patients respectively receiving 1 and 5 mg of DES. These results suggest that endocrine therapy **effectively improves sur-**

vival rates at least in patients with stage D prostatic cancer.

Lepor et al. (1982) compared the survival of 654 stage C and D patients treated during the pre-endocrine period (1937-1940) with a similar group treated by hormones between 1942 and 1943. The study was designed to minimise the influence of general medical progress on patient survival. The mean survival for the group treated during the pre-endocrine period was 530 days compared with 709 days in the patients receiving endocrine therapy. This difference was statistically significant but the possible influence of a natural increase in longevity during this post-endocrine period could not be excluded.

2. Are oestrogens more effective than castration ?

Another erroneous conclusion of the VACURG studies was based on the concept that **oestrogens were more effective than castration in the reduction of mortality from prostatic cancer** (Blackard et al., 1973). This concept was based on a poor interpretation of the first study in which the patients treated with oestrogens had the lowest cancer mortality rate. In fact, since the patients treated with oestrogens had an excessive cardiovascular mortality essentially occurring during the first year of treatment, it is probable that many of these patients would have died from cancer if they had not died from cardiovascular causes during the first year of endocrine therapy. In a study by Nesbit and Baum (1950), the 5-year survival of patients with stage D cancer was 10% for those receiving 1 to 5 mg of DES, 22% for those treated with castration alone and 20% for those treated by the two modalities. This suggests that castration is the most effective form and that the administration of 1 to 5 mg of DES to castrated patients did not improve survival. Overall, adequate oestrogen therapy, or castration, appear to provide equivalent results and there is little to be gained from combining the two modalities.

Castration is preferred because it is a more reliable, though more radical method of ensuring adequate suppression of plasma testosterone, avoiding the problems of patient compliance reported in several papers. For example, it has been demonstrated that testosterone levels could return to normal levels within twelve hours if the dose of 1 mg of DES per day was not taken (Beck et al., 1978).

In another report (1977), Michigan and Catalona treated patients with ureteric obstruction by endocrine therapy. Of the castrated patients, 88% had a favourable response compared with 17% of those treated with DES or with an antiandrogen, cyproterone acetate.

IV. COMPLICATIONS OF DES

Although widely used in the treatment of metastatic prostatic cancer, the clinical value of DES has been a controversial subject over recent years since the VACURG group (Veterans administration Cooperative Urological Research Group) drew attention to the cardiovascular complications, particularly thromboembolic, which can cancel out the benefit obtained by this treatment on the cancer itself. Hypertensive crises and salt and water retention were also reported.

The thromboembolic cardiovascular complications associated with oestrogen therapy for prostatic cancer are related to fluid retention, alteration of plasma antithrombin III levels, increased platelet aggregation and changes in plasma lipids. Antithrombin III is an $\alpha2$-globulin produced by the liver which seems to be the most important physiological inhibitor of coagulation. Some studies have shown that the administration of oestrogen decreases the levels of antithrombin III to zones of hypercoagulability. Patients undergoing castration have normal antithrombin III levels. DES (15 mg per day) markedly decreases the levels of antithrombin III in the plasma, while patients receiving only 1 mg of DES per day have normal antithrombin III levels.

The increased platelet aggregation can be largely prevented by the use of aspirin.

Other side effects of administration of DES, such as feminisation, decreased libido, impotence, azoospermia, gastrointestinal disturbances, nausea and vomiting, have also been reported. However, these side effects are dose-dependent and are minimal with a dose of 1 mg of DES per day, but this low dose does not completely suppress testicular activity and the plasma testosterone concentration may rise to above castrate levels at certain times during the day. The dose of 2 mg may be ideal both in terms of efficacy and limitation of the complications, but no studies have been conducted with this dose to date.

V. OESTROGENS OTHER THAN DES.

Oestrogens other than DES have been used for the treatment of disseminated prostatic cancer but none can be considered to have achieved universal acceptance. The long-acting *polyoestradiol phosphate* (Estradurin) is popular in Scandinavia. It is injected intramuscularly (80-160 mg/month), it only weakly suppresses LH secretion. *Premarin* (2.5 mg t.d.s.), a mixture of conjugated equine oestrogens, and *ethinyloestradiol-17β* (0.15-1.0 mg/day), are generally considered to be less effective and more expensive than DES.

DOCUMENTATION

MELLINGER, G.T. Veterans Administration Cooperative Urological Research Group. Carcinoma of the prostate: A continuing co-operative study. J. Urol. 91, 1964, 500-594.

ARDUINO, L.J. Veterans Administration Cooperative Urological Research Group. Carcinoma of the prostate: Treatment and comparisons. J. Urol. 98, 1967, 516-522.

BYAR, D.P. VACURG studies on prostatic cancer and its treatment. In: Urological Pathology: The Prostate. (Tannenbaum, M., Ed.) New York, Lea and Febiger, 1977, pp 241-267.

Surgical Castration

S. Khoury

Department of Urology, Hôpital de la Pitié, Paris, France

I. HORMONAL CONSEQUENCES

90% of the circulating testosterone is derived from the testes. Bilateral castration decreases the plasma testosterone level from 500 ng per 100 ml to about 50 ng per 100 ml in the great majority of cases (Plate 1).

II. TECHNIQUE

1. Castration (Plate 2)

Anaesthesia : General, or preferably local anaesthesia can be used. The technique for local anaesthesia is described in Plate 1.

Bilateral castration is generally performed via two inguinal incisions or a horizontal infrapubic incision.

Testicular prostheses may be inserted at the end of the operation when desired by the patient.

2. Pulpectomy (Plate 2)

Pulpectomy consists of removing the secretory pulp of the testis, while leaving the albuginea, which is closed.

3. Extra-epididymal castration (Plate 2)

This operation achieves the same cosmetic effect as pulpectomy and would appear to be preferable, as it avoids the risk of leaving behind a few islands of Leydig cells.

III. RESULTS

Castration gives results equivalent to those of oestrogen without the disadvantages of metabolic and cardiovascular complications and feminisation.

However, impotence is the general rule after castration, although some patients continue to have a certain degree of sexual activity. The comparative results have already been discussed in the chapter on oestrogens.

Surgical castration should be preferred to the use of oestrogens. However, more and more, it is tending to be replaced by LHRH analogues, which do not have the psychological disadvantages of castration.

The use of LHRH analogues will almost certainly replace surgical castration in the future, especially when sustained-release injections (3 to 6 months) become available at a lower price.

DOCUMENTATION

KAYE KW. Infrapubic operations : Vasovasostomy and bilateral orchiectomy. In Outpatient Urologic Surgery. Lea et Febiger. 1985, 217.

MACKLER MA et al. The effect of orchiectomy and various doses of stilbestrol on plasma testosterone levels in patients with carcinoma of the prostate. Invest. Urol, 1972, 9, 423-425.

O'CONNOR VJ, CHIANG SP, GRAYHACK JT. Is subcapsular orchiectomy a definitive procedure? Studies of hormone excretion before and after orchiectomy. J. Urol., 1963, 89, 236-240.

Surgical castration: Hormonal consequences

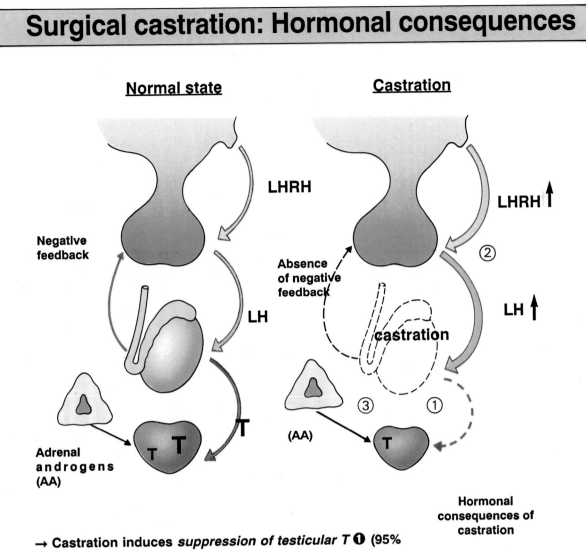

Normal state

LHRH

Negative feedback

LH

T

T T

Adrenal androgens (AA)

Castration

LHRH ↑

②

Absence of negative feedback

castration

LH ↑

(AA)

③   ①

T

→ Castration induces *suppression of testicular T* ❶ (95% of plasma T). This results in a *reactive rise* in LHRH and LH. ❷

→ The 5% of circulating T which persists is derived from the *adrenal glands.*❸

According to some authors, this marked fall in plasma T is not accompanied by a similar fall in intraprostatic DHT, which remains at about 30% of its initial value (by metabolism of adrenal androgens). This would allow cancer cells very sensitive to DHT to continue to proliferate despite castration. This explains the value, for these authors, of *combined androgenic blockade* which would also block the action of adrenal androgens.

Hormonal consequences of castration

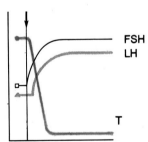

FSH
LH

T

Castration : Technique

I. CASTRATION

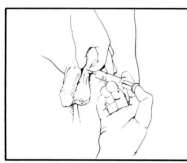

Figure 1. General, or preferably local anaesthesia can be used.Anaesthetic block of the spermatic cord when the cord can be pinched between the index finger and the thumb.

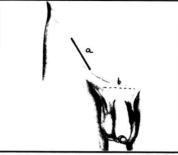

Figure 2. Castration : Incisions :
a) Inguinal incision,
b) Infrapubic incision.

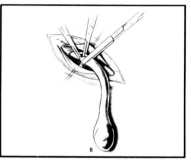

Figure 3. The cord is divided into two segments which are then ligated separately.

II. PULPECTOMY

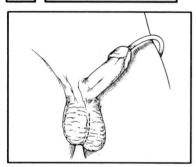

Figure 4. Scrotal incision.
a) Midline
b) Separate

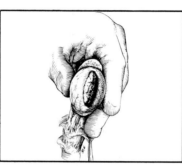

Figure 5. Incision of the tunica albuginea in the axis of the testicle.

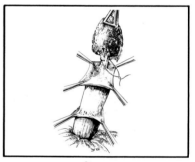

Figure 6. The seminiferous tubules and vessels located in the head of the epididymis form a pedicle which is clamped and ligated on mass by a heavy ligature. Cauterisation with an electric scalpel of the internal surface.

III. EXTRA-EPIDIDYMAL CASTRATION

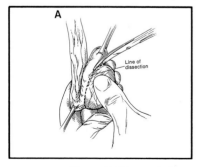

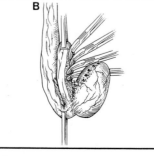

Figure 7. The testis is separated from the epididymis.

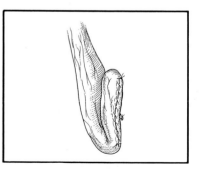

Figure 8. The epididymis is sutured onto itself. Final appearance.

LHRH Analogues

S. Khoury

Department of Urology, Hôpital de la Pitié, Paris, France

The LHRH analogues goserelin (Zoladex)*, leuprolide, tryptorelin and buserelin are registered in many countries for the treatment of prostate cancer. Being peptides, they are susceptible to digestion in the gastrointestinal tract and therefore other routes of administration need to be used to establish sustained plasma concentrations.

Injections, which have to be given daily, and nasal sprays, which must be taken several times a day, may be less convenient and reliable than *longer acting depot preparations.* Three of these analogues are available in such depot formulations, 'Zoladex', leuprolide and tryptorelin, for administration every 28 days. Serum testosterone concentrations are suppressed to the castrate range by 3-4 weeks after the initial administration, and remain suppressed provided the drugs are given on a *monthly basis*.

Following the original work of Huggins in 1941, *orchidectomy* and *oestrogens* have become the standard endocrine approach to the palliative treatment of advanced prostatic cancer.

The introduction of *LHRH analogues* has provided an *alternative medical approach* to the treatment of prostate cancer avoiding surgery and its potential complications or the risk of the cardiovascular side effects of oestrogen therapy.

---

* 'Zoladex' is a trade mark, the property of Imperial Chemical Industries PLC.

LHRH analogues and antagonists

1. LHRH

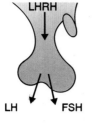

Definition

LHRH is the hypothalamic hormone responsible for stimulation of hypophyseal gonadotrope cells. It stimulates the secretion of two gonadotrophins, FSH and LH. However, its effects are more marked on LH than on FSH, which has led some authors to question the existence of a specific FSH releasing factor.

Structure

LHRH has an identical structure in all mammals : it is a decapeptide formed by a chain of 10 amino acids which forms a C-shaped configuration in aqueous solution.

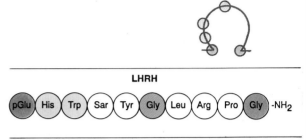

LHRH

pGlu – His – Trp – Sar – Tyr – Gly – Leu – Arg – Pro – Gly – -NH₂

2. LHRH analogues

Definition

LHRH agonists have a very similar structure to natural LHRH. They reversibly inhibit the production of sex steroids.

Structural modifications

The synthesis of LHRH agonists requires **structural modifications** in order to increase the lifespan of the compound and to **increase its affinity** for the receptor, therefore resulting in more potent peptides with a longer duration of action.

LHRH AGONISTS EVALUATED BY CLINICAL TRIALS IN PROSTATIC CANCER

LHRH	1 Pyro-Glu	2 His	3 Trp	4 Ser	5 Tyrr	6 Gly	7 Leu	8 Arg	9 Pro	10 Glu-NH₂
D-Trp 6-LHRH						D-Trp				
Buserelin						D-Ser (tBU)				Ethylamide
Leuprolide						D-Leu				Ethylamide
Goserelin						D-Ser (tBU)				Az-Gly -NH₂

The **glycine in the 6** position is the site of proteolytic attack : agonists have been synthesised by replacing this residue by a dextrogyral amino acid, which increases the stability of the molecule and increases its binding affinity. This substitution decreases the sensitivity to proteolysis and increases the biological activity. These peptides are therefore **more potent than natural LHRH** (50-100 times). The table opposite summarises the principal LHRH agonists used clinically in prostatic cancer.

3. LHRH antagonists

Conversely, modifications of the first amino acids (principally replacement of histidine in position (2) induces an antagonist activity: the molecules bind to LHRH receptors and block them without exerting any biological activity.

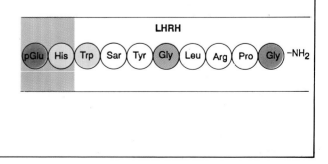

LHRH

pGlu – His – Trp – Sar – Tyr – Gly – Leu – Arg – Pro – Gly – -NH₂

Mechanism of action of LHRH analogues

1. Physiological action

LHRH is secreted by the hypothalamus and is released directly into the capillaries, reaching the anterior pituitary via the hypothalamo-hypophyseal portal system to act directly on the gonadotrope cells of the antehypophysis. LHRH binds specifically to membrane receptors situated on the surface of pituitary gonadotrope cells. The binding of LHRH to its receptor triggers the secretion of LH and FSH.

Regulation of LHRH receptors.

LHRH receptors only retain their activity while they are intermittently occupied, which is normally the case, as LHRH is secreted according to a pulsatile mode and has a short half-life.

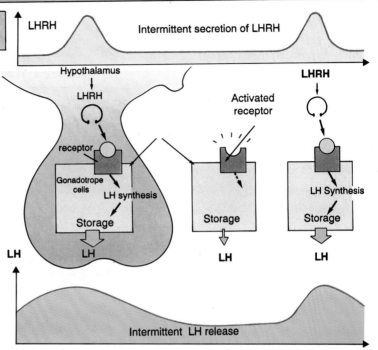

2. Continuous administration

On the other hand, when the receptors are continuously occupied by LHRH perfusion or by an agonist, the hypophyseal gonadotrope receptors become desensitized resulting in inhibition of gonadotrophin secretion 10 to 15 days later. This results in a marked fall in LH and FSH secretion. Furthermore, the number of LHRH receptors decreases secondarily during "desensitization".

This phenomenon is the *basis* for the *clinical use of LHRH agonists.*

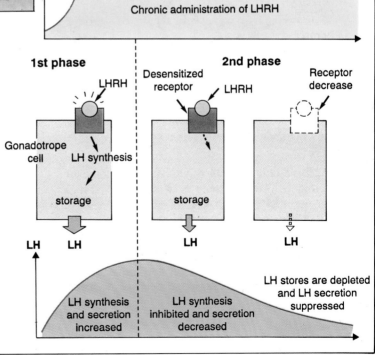

3. Action of LHRH analogues

LHRH analogues have a similar but much more potent action than natural LHRH.

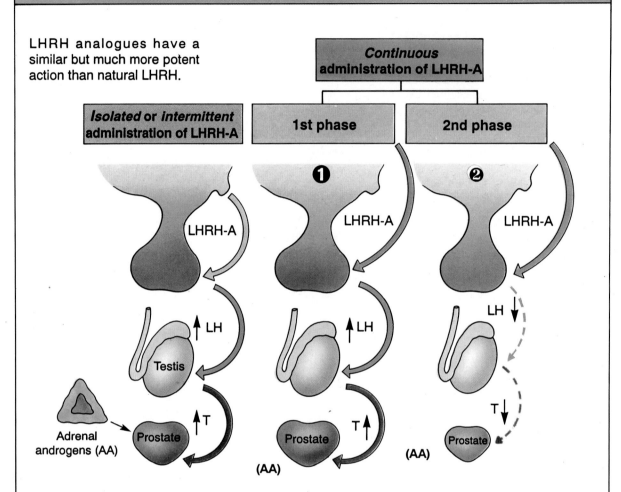

Continuous administration of LHRH-A

Isolated or **intermittent** administration of LHRH-A

1st phase

2nd phase

→ Isolated or intermittent administration of LHRH analogues, as under physiological conditions, induces an increased secretion of LH and testosterone. ❶

→ A biphasic phenomenon occurs during continuous administration : initially, there is a rise in LH and T (flare-up), as in ❶, followed, several days later, by a fall in LH and testosterone levels which reach castration levels after 3 to 4 weeks ❷. LHRH analogues do not affect the adrenal secretion of testosterone.

This effect is due to desensitization and rarefaction of hypophyseal receptors by large and continuous doses of LHRH analogues.

Hormonal consequences of _prolonged administration_ of LHRH analogues

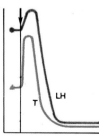

Hot flushes: mechanism and prevention

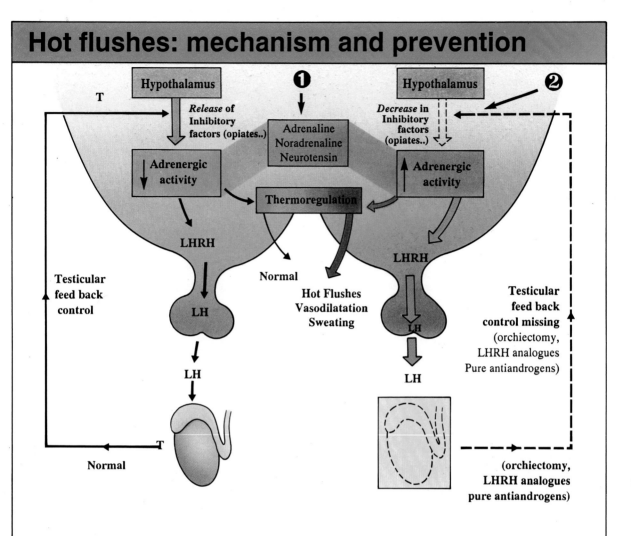

It is well known that hot flushes are somehow attached to the **neuroendocrine counterregulation mechanism** induced by low sex-steroid levels. Recent findings have shown that not the rise in gonadotrophins, but **high hypothalamic concentrations of norepinephrine (NE)** are the reason for hot flushes. NE is the neurotransmitter for LHRH and is therefore involved in the central counter-regulatory process.

Sex-steroids stimulate the release of substances (probably opioids) which inhibit NE release. A sharp decrease in the sex-steroid level, caused by orchiectomy or LHRH agonists, results in a **failure to inhibit NE**. Consequently, an excessive NE release occurs and disturbs the central thermoregulation. The clinical result of this disturbance is **hot flushes**.

Prevention of hot flushes is possible with substances which:

a) **block NE centrally** (e.g.; Clonidine) ❶ or,

b) which **reinstate the release of inhibitory opioids** (e.g., androgens, œstrogens, and progestogens).❷

This explains why antiandrogens with additional progestogenic activity, such as CPA, have a positive therapeutic effect on hot flushes in orchiectomized patients or patients treated with LHRH agonists.

"Flare-up"

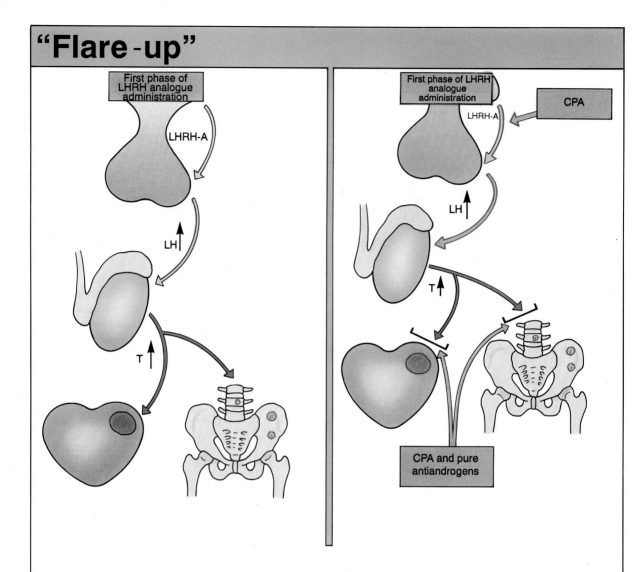

After administration of LHRH analogues, an ***initial elevation of LH and testosterone*** is followed after 1 to 2 weeks by a ***gradual inhibition, bringing testosterone to castrate levels***. This
transient elevation of serum testosterone ***may initially stimulate tumour growth*** (flare reac-
tion), and up to 10% of patients experience exacerbation of pain symptoms. To avoid such complications, an ***antiandrogen*** is sometimes administered concurrently with an LHRH analogue
during the first month of treatment.

During this phase, the central and peripheral inhibitory effect of cyproterone acetate effectively
blocks the "flare-up" phenomenon. Jacobi treated 23 patients with an LHRH analogue together
with cyproterone acetate (150 mg/day) and found no significant stimulation of serum testosterone. Similar results were obtained by Boccon-Gibod et al. ***Pure antiandrogens*** act by blocking
the testosterone action on target tumour cells.

Clinical Studies with LHRH Analogues

S. Khoury

Department of Urology, Hôpital de la Pitié, Paris, France

1. Treatment of advanced disease

a) Clinical studies

A large number of **non-comparative studies** have been reported with LHRH analogues in patients with prostate cancer.

However, as far as **phase III trials** are concerned, only, **'Zoladex'** ® * (goserelin) has been compared with both orchidectomy and oestrogens in large randomised studies (Kaisary et al., 1991; Waymont et al., 1992; Kuhn et al., 1990). **Buserelin** has been compared with a combined group of stilboestrol or orchidectomy treated patients (Klioze et al., 1988); **leuprolide** with oestrogens (The Leuprolide Study Group., 1988; ASO et al., 1991); and **tryptorelin** (Parmar et al., 1988; De Sy et al., 1988) with orchidectomy. In these studies, no statistically significant differences have been found between LHRH analogue therapy and either orchidectomy or oestrogens as far as objective response rate and overall survival are concerned.

In the 'Zoladex' versus stilboestrol study, the median time to first response was more rapid for 'Zoladex'. However, the median time to treatment failure was shorter for buserelin than for DES/orchidectomy (Klioze et al., 1988).

A wealth of **side effects** has been reported in the stilboestrol treated patients in these studies, particularly cardiovascular effects and gynaecomastia. Indeed, almost half of the 36

---

* 'Zoladex' is a trade mark, the property of Imperial Chemical Industries PLC.

Table 1. Randomised comparative studies of LHRH agonists with orchidectomy or with œstrogens.

Objective response		
'Zoladex' n = 148 71%	Orchidectomy n = 144 72%	Kaisary A.V. et al., 1991
Tryptorelin n = 55 83%	Orchidectomy n = 58 82%	Parmar H. et al., 1988
Tryptorelin n = 40 68%	Orchidectomy n = 16 71%	De Sy W.A. et al., 1988
(results at 12 months)		
'Zoladex' n = 124 71%	Stilboestrol n = 126 57%	Waymont et al., 1992
Leuprolide (daily injection) n = 92 86%	Stilboestrol n = 94 85%	The Leuprolide Study Group 1988
'Zoladex' n = 107 87%	Estracyt n = 95 95%	Kuhn et al., 1990
Leuprolide n = 66 55%	Fosfestrol n = 68 47%	Aso et al., 1991
(criteria of the Jap. Cancer Study Group)		
Buserelin n = 105 63%	DES/Orchidectomy n = 41 n = 14 65%	Klioze et al., 1988

withdrawals in the DES group were due to cardiovascular effects in the 'Zoladex' stilboestrol comparison (Waymont et al., 1992).

In the LHRH analogue groups, the reported side effects have been mainly those expected from the pharmacological effects of **testosterone suppression**, such as hot flushes, loss of libido and impotence. Some initial increases in bone pain in patients with bone metastases have been observed which are thought to result from the initial rise in serum testosterone caused by these drugs, although the incidence has been low (less than 5%). Serious complications, such as ureteric obstruction and spinal cord compression, which have been associated with the disease process also, have been reported.

b) The patient's choice

Clinicians are becoming increasingly aware that patient choice is an important aspect of treatment and its success. Of **2 studies** in which patients with advanced disease were given a choice between 'Zoladex' or orchidectomy as their initial treatment, 78% of 147 and 86% of 57 patients, respectively, chose 'Zoladex' (Cassileth et al., 1989; Lunglmayr et al., 1987). The main reasons for this choice were the avoidance of surgery and cosmetic factors. In the larger of the studies, when asked again three months later, 93% of the patients and 91% of their wives indicated that they would select the same treatment.

2. Down-staging in localised disease

More recently, a possible role for LHRH analogues has been suggested in the treatment of non-metastatic prostate cancer. Given usually for **3 months prior** to a **prostatectomy** or **radiotherapy,** shrinkage of the prostate tumour has been reported (Pilepich et al., 1990; Flamm et al., 1991).

In conclusion, comparative studies in advanced prostate cancer have shown that LHRH analogues provide a **generally well tolerated medical alternative to standard therapy** such as surgical castration.

DOCUMENTATION

KAISARY AV., TYRRELL CJ., PEELING WB., GRIFFITHS K. : Comparison of LHRH analogue ('Zoladex') with orchiectomy in patients with metastatic prostatic carcinoma. Br.J.Urol.67 :502-508, 1991.

PARMAR H., PHILLIPS RH., LIGHTMAN SL., EDWARDS L. : How would you like to have an orchidectomy for advanced prostatic cancer? Am.J.Clin.Oncol.II :S160-S168, 1988

DE SY WA., DE WILDE P., DE MEYER JM., CASSELMAN J., DESMET R., RENDERS G., SCHELFHOUT W. : Long term experience in the treatment of advanced prostatic cancer with decapeptyl, compared to orchidectomy. Acta.Urologica.Belgica.56 :581-587, 1988

WAYMONT B., LYNCH TH., DUNN JA., EMTAGE LA., ARKELL DG., WALLACE DMA., BLACKLEDGE GRP. : Phase III randomised study of 'Zoladex' versus stilboestrol in the treatment of advanced prostate cancer. Br.J.Urol.69 :614-620, 1992

THE LEUPROLIDE STUDY GROUP. : Leuprolide versus diethylstilbestrol for metastatic prostate cancer. N.Eng.J.Med.311 :1281-1286, 1988

KUHN MW., WEIBACH L. : Primary therapy of metastasized carcinoma of the prostate with 'Zoladex' versus estracyt-preliminary report. Recent. Adv. Urol. Cancers. Diagnosis. Treatment :86-89, 1990

KLIOZE SS., MILLER MF., SPIRO TP. : A randomized, comparative study of buserelin with DES/orchiectomy in the treatment of stage D2 prostatic cancer patients. Am.J.Clin.Oncol.II :S176-S182, 1988

ASO Y., KAMEYAMA S., NIIJIMA T., OHMORI H., OHIASHI T., ET AL. : Clinical phase III study on TAP-144-SR, an LHRH agonist depot formulation, in patients with prostatic cancer. Hinyokika.Kiyo.37 :305-320, 1991

CASSILETH BR., SOLOWAY MS., VOGELZANG NJ., SCHELLHAMMER PS., SEIDMON EJ., HAIT HI., KENNEALEY GT. : Patients' choice of treatment in stage D prostate cancer. Suppl.Urol.XXXIII :57-62, 1989

LUNGLMAYR G., GIRSCH E., BIEGLMAYER CH. : Acceptability of orchidectomy versus GNRH-agonists in the management of advanced cancer of the prostate. J.Endocrinol.Invest.10 :20, 1987

PILEPICH MV., JOHN MJ., KRALL JM., MCGOWEN D., HWONG YS., PERIZ CA STUDY GROUP. : Phase III radiation therapy oncology group study of hormonal cytoreduction with flutamide and 'Zoladex' in locally advanced carcinoma of the prostate treated with definitive radiotherapy. Am J Clin Oncol.13 :461-464, 1990

FLAMM J., FISCHER M., HOELTL W., PFLUERGER H., TOMSCHI W. : Complete androgen deprivation prior to radical prostatectomy in patients with stage T3 cancer of the prostate. Eur.Urol.19 :192-195

Antiandrogens

S. Khoury

Department of Urology, Hôpital de la Pitié, Paris, France

At present there are two fundamentally different types of antiandrogen.

One group comprises **non-steroidal substances.** Apart from their antiandrogenic property, they are devoid of other hormonal activity; they are therefore also known as **pure antiandrogens** (e.g. flutamide, nilutamide).

The other group consists of **steroidal antiandrogens** : In addition to their antiandrogenic effects, they also display progestational and, closely associated with this, **antigonadotrophic properties** (e.g. cyproterone acetate, megesterone acetate, chlormadione acetate).

In general, antiandrogens are well tolerated by the patient. Common to all antiandrogens, especially the pure antiandrogens, is their **better cardiovascular tolerance** compared with traditional oestrogen therapy.

Despite the differences in structure, the **antiandrogenic effect** of all known compounds is based on an identical molecular mechanism. They **compete with androgens** for the **binding sites at the androgen receptor** in the nucleus of target cells. Their therapeutic efficacy is therefore assured only when the ratio of antiandrogens to androgens is maintained at a sufficiently high level - i.e. in excess.

However, there are important differences between the two types of antiandrogen in *in vivo* use. The reason for this is the presence and absence, respectively, of antigonadotrophic activity.

Their mechanism of action and their interaction with the endocrine regulatory system will be summarised in the following plates.

DOCUMENTATION

NEUMANN F., BORMARCHER K. Differences in action and toxicity of antiandrogens In: Murphy GP, Khoury S., (eds). Therapeutic Progress in Urological Cancers, pages 123-128. Alan R. Liss, New York 1989.

KENNEALEY G., FURR B.J.A. Use of the nonsteroidal anti-androgen casodex in advanced prostatic cancer. Urologic clinics of North America 18, N01, 99-110, 1991

Antiandrogens

1. Definition and mechanism of action

In order to elicit their biological action androgens (DHT) must be selectively bound to a nuclear androgen Receptor (AR). Binding to AR conditions DHT action.

Antiandrogens inhibit the effect of androgens at the target cells, by competing with them for the androgen receptor binding sites. Unlike the **Androgen**- AR complex, the **Antiandrogen**-AR complex is unable to interact with the chromatin and thus does not promote the androgen mediated gene regulatory processes.

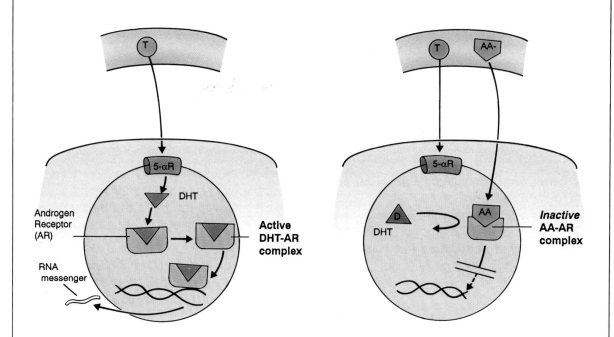

There are two families of antiandrogen :

- **Pure antiandrogens** with no antigonadotrophic action (Flutamide, Nilutanide , "Casodex"*)

- **Steroidal antiandrogens** with both antiandrogenic and antigonadotrophic (progestational) properties (Cyproterone Acetate)

These two types behave differently *in vivo*

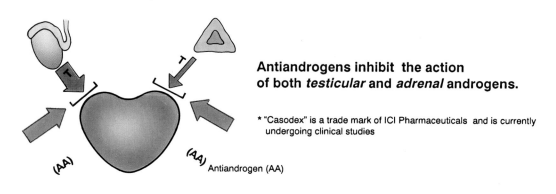

Antiandrogens inhibit the action of both *testicular* and *adrenal* androgens.

* "Casodex" is a trade mark of ICI Pharmaceuticals and is currently undergoing clinical studies

Antiandrogen (AA)

Steroidal antiandrogens

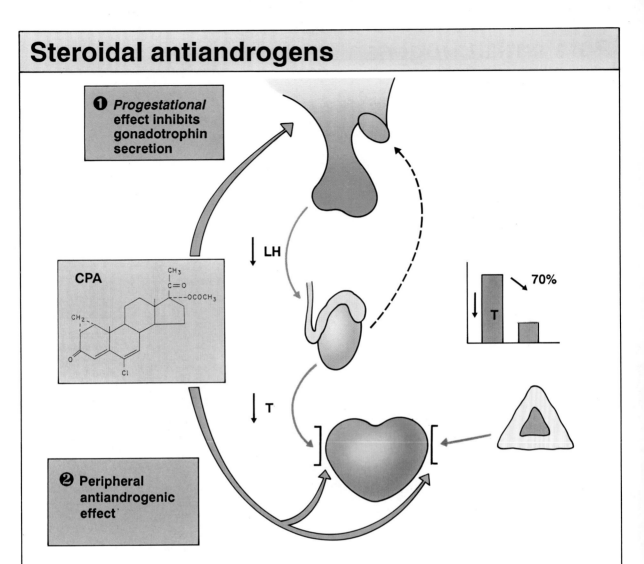

❶ *Progestational* effect inhibits gonadotrophin secretion

CPA

↓ LH

↓ T

70%

T

❷ Peripheral antiandrogenic effect

Steroidal antiandrogens such as cyproterone acetate (CPA) and megesterol acetate are *progestational* as well as being *antiandrogenic*, restraining the effect of DHT within the prostate and simultaneously *decreasing gonadotrophin secretion*, thereby lowering the concentration of testosterone in plasma to "subcastrate" levels.

An EORTC Phase III trial subsequently compared 3 mg/d DES, with CPA (250 mg/d) and also with medroxyprogesterone acetate (MPA 200 mg/d), as primary endocrine therapy for advanced disease. It was reported that, with respect to "time to disease progression" and survival, *CPA and DES were equally effective*, with cardiovascular problems twice as prevalent with DES than CPA ; *MPA was less clinically effective* than either DES or CPA.

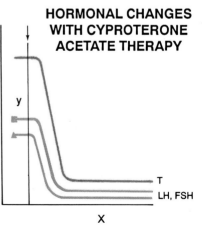

HORMONAL CHANGES WITH CYPROTERONE ACETATE THERAPY

y

T

LH, FSH

X

Pure antiandrogens

1. Mechanism of action

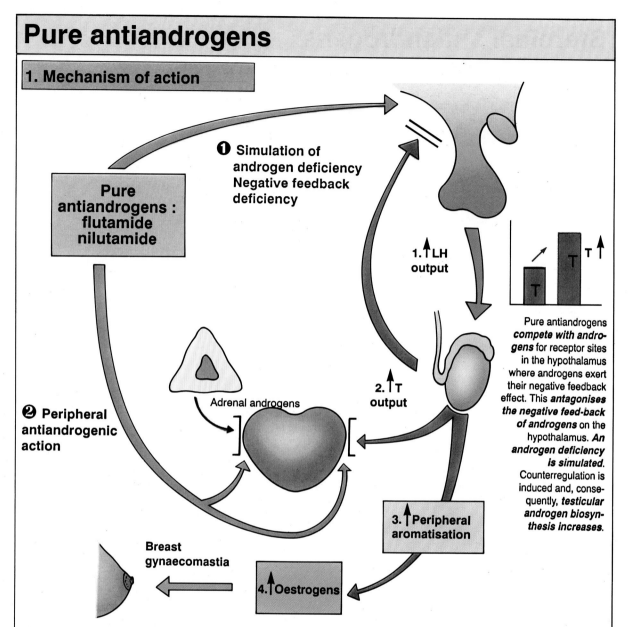

❶ Simulation of androgen deficiency Negative feedback deficiency

Pure antiandrogens : flutamide nilutamide

1. ↑ LH output

2. ↑ T output

❷ Peripheral antiandrogenic action

Adrenal androgens

3. ↑ Peripheral aromatisation

4. ↑ Oestrogens

Breast gynaecomastia

Pure antiandrogens *compete with androgens* for receptor sites in the hypothalamus where androgens exert their negative feedback effect. This *antagonises the negative feed-back of androgens* on the hypothalamus. *An androgen deficiency is simulated.* Counterregulation is induced and, consequently, *testicular androgen biosynthesis increases.*

Flutamide and *nilutamide* are pure antiandrogens. They have marked effects, not only within the prostate, but also at the level of the hypothalamic-pituitary axis where androgens normally elicit a negative feedback control on the release of LH. This leads to an increased LH output and a subsequent *increase in the synthesis and secretion of testosterone*, with Leydig cell hyperplasia. The increased peripheral aromatisation of testoterone results in an *increased plasma concentration of oestradiol* and painful gynaecomastia.

Casodex (ICI 176, 334) is a new, non-steroidal pure antiandrogen under development which has the advantage of a relatively *long half-life,* allowing once-daily dosing.

Since the inhibiton at the receptor is competitive, the increased amount of testoterone *can abolish either completely or partly the antiandrogenic effect of these short half-life pure antiandrogens* after a certain period of time. This explains why spermatogenesis and libido are not or only partially inhibited. This possibility has influenced the decision to use these pure antiandrogens as a *primary endocrine monotherapy* for prostatic cancer. They are, however, extensively *used in combination with LHRH analogues or castration* for the treatment of advanced prostatic cancer .

Estramustine Phosphate

S. Khoury
Department of Urology, Hôpital de la Pitié, Paris, France

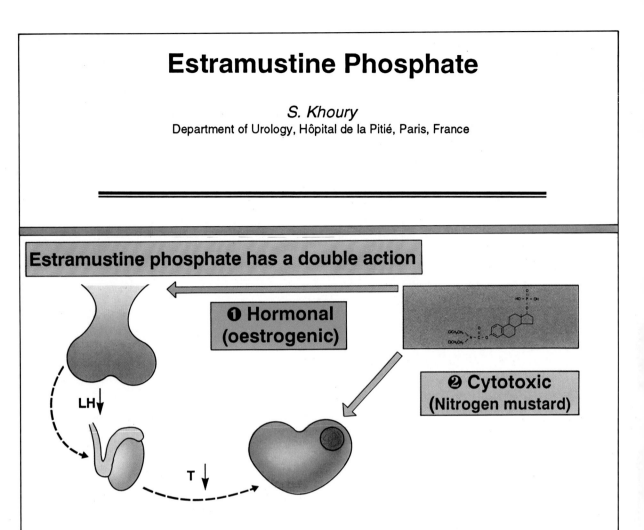

Estramustine phosphate has a double action

❶ Hormonal (oestrogenic)

❷ Cytotoxic (Nitrogen mustard)

LH↓

T↓

Estramustine was introduced in the clinical treatment of prostate cancer by Konyves in 1966. It is a molecule that combines chemically *oestradiol* and *nitrogen mustard* with a *carbamate linkage*. It is presented as a phosphate to make it soluble.

Being a compound that is both *oestrogenic and cytotoxic*, the **main indication** of this drug is second or third line treatment in prostate cancer patients resistant to hormonal therapy. In hormone-refractory patients, the response rate is 30% objective, with 40% subjective improvement for a mean duration of 5 months.

It is also indicated as a **primary treatment** in disseminated prostatic cancer of poor prognosis (very undifferentiated tumours, young patients).

Side effects are mainly those of oestrogens. Bone marrow failure due to the nitrogen mustard is very rare. When it occurs, treatment should be stopped till recovery. Periodic blood counts are usually needed (once every two months).

Choice of Primary Treatment

S. Khoury

Department of Urology, Hôpital de la Pitié, Paris, France

The most direct technique for lowering plasma androgen levels is **bilateral orchidectomy,** removing the primary source of testosterone in male patients for a lifetime. This simple surgery decreases tissue DHT levels to 20% of their preoperative value: ± 4 pmol/g of tissue in most patients.

Medical castration was achieved previous decades by the oral administration of 5 mg **diethylstilboestrol (DES)** daily. A number of studies from VACURG and EORTC confirmed its efficacy for cancer control but revealed significant **cardiovascular toxicity and associated mortality.**

Most authors agree that medical castration is probably better achieved today by the depot administration of **long-acting LHRH analogues**. Randomised trials have shown that these drugs are as effective as orchidectomy or DES 3 mg daily. This efficacy was again confirmed in an open randomized trial. The safety record of the LHRH analogues is good and in patients receiving long-term treatment have confirmed the lasting treatment efficacy. This excellent track record prompted the search for 3-monthly formulations which are now undergoing clinical evaluation. The physiological surge of testosterone induced by the initial LHRH analogues administration can be countered by the administration of an anti-androgen given for 1 week prior to LHRH agonist and continued during the first month of therapy.

Medical castration by LHRH analogues therapy will almost certainly replace surgical castration in the future.

Table 1. The selection of primary endocrine treatment.

	Patient's preferences	Treatment choice
Good prognostic factors	Preserve sexuality	Watchful waiting Pure antiandrogens
	Indifferent sexual status	LHRH-A Surgical castration
Poor prognostic factors		LHRH-A Surgical castration Maximal androgen blockade

Antiandrogens have been given as monotherapy in small studies, but generally in combination with either surgical or medical castration. They are effective in blocking the "flare-up" phenomenon induced by LHRH analogues.

The continuous addition of antiandrogens to castration (surgical or medical) forms the regimen for **combination treatment** (maximal androgen blockade). The aim is to attempt to **block the adrenal** and **testicular androgens**. The results of randomised trials using combination treatment showed conflicting results and a meta-analysis of 17 randomised studies is awaited to show if survival and/or quality of life is enhanced by the initiation of combination treatment.

DOCUMENTATION

DENIS L. Current strategies in hormonal manipulation of advanced prostate cancer. Current Opinion in Urology 1991, 1:16-20.

Early Versus Delayed Hormonal Treatment

S. Khoury

Department of Urology, Hôpital de la Pitié, Paris, France

A number of recent studies have generated renewed interest in the concept of immediate androgen deprivation.

Early therapy delays the onset of disease progression and improves survival in a certain category of patients.

The concept that asymptomatic patients with prostate cancer could benefit from deferred treatment at the time of onset of symptoms is based on the publication of the Veterans Administration Cooperative Urological Research Group (VACURG).

However, a critical review and reanalysis of these results in patients with stage C and stage D showed that younger patients with stage D disease and high-grade tumours (Gleason score 7-10) derive a survival benefit from early therapy.

Furthermore, it is well established that early androgen ablation will markedly delay the onset of disease progression in the majority of treated patients. Moreover, the patient will enjoy the benefits of a longer symptom-free interval, which logically correlates with an improved quality of life. Obviously, these benefits are substantial, and many urologists find them sufficiently compelling to recommend early hormonal therapy. Although somewhat empirical, this approach seems justifiable for several reasons.

a) Morbidity has decreased with new alternatives.

Morbidity of hormonal treatment was an argument in favour of delayed treatment. Today, although not insignificant, the morbidity associated with androgen deprivation therapy has decreased substantially with the advent of effective pharmacological alternatives to DES (Long-acting LHRH analogues).

b) Theoretical experimental evidence concerning tumour progression tends to favour early treatment.

Finally, there are a number of theoretical benefits to be derived from early hormonal therapy. Because of the impact of genetic instability, there appears to be a trend toward increasing aneuploidy and androgen resistance as the tumour volume increases. Thus, delaying androgen ablation **could promote the development of additional androgen-resistant clones**, rendering subsequent therapy more problematic. Conversely, early androgen deprivation would permit the initiation of therapy in a relatively vigorous patient with a good performance level. The prompt identification of nonresponders in that group would facilitate the use of additional cystostatic or cytotoxic therapies because:

1. such treatment is generally more effective when directed against small tumour burdens.

2. patients with a good performance level (i.e., manageable tumour burdens) are more likely to tolerate and benefit from aggressive systemic therapy. Thus, the cytoreductive impact of androgen ablation might induce the recruitment of androgen-insensitive cells from G0 into more active phases of the cell cycle and so render them more susceptible to cytotoxic therapy.

c) The discussion between early and deferred hormonal treatment is rather theoretical. In practice, the great majority of candidates for hormonal treatment are advanced cases and already have a certain degree of symptoms that cannot be left untreated without affecting the patient's quality of life.

Conclusion : The risk benefit analysis is strongly ***in favour of early hormonal therapy.***

DOCUMENTATION

KOZLOWSKI J.M., ELLIS W.J., GRAYHACK J.T.
  Advanced prostatic cancer: Early versus late endocrine therapy. Urol Clin North Am 18, 1, 1991

Should Hormonal Therapy be Stopped After Relapse Following Primary Hormonal Treatment ?

S. Khoury

Urology Department, Hôpital de la Pitié, Paris, France

The increasing use of reversible medical castration (LHRH analogues, antiandrogens) raises the question of whether hormonal therapy should be stopped in the event of escape from the treament.

The outlook for patients failing hormone therapy is poor. However, nowhere in the literature is there a categorical statement to the effect that this ineffective and failing therapy should be stopped, and there is a lack of information on what would happen to patients if this were routinely practised and the results recorded. It is implied in the literature, though not stated, that therapy is continued despite progression of the disease and it is obviously correct to question why this should be so. In fact, there is often great resistance by clinicians to the cessation of therapy for 3 main reasons :

1. The resistance to a specific endocrine treatment does not imply that **all cancer cells are hormone independent,** since the administration of **exogenous testosterone still provokes exacerbation of tumour growth** in the great majority of cases.

2. There is the **fear of an accelerated relapse** when the androgen deprivation therapy is removed allowing the hormonally-sensitive clone to grow again. However for the investigator who fears an accelerated relapse, orchidectomy is available to ensure castrate testosterone levels, provided the patient accepts this and is fit enough for the operation.

This is the recommendation made by the EORTC Genitourinary Group for patients entered into the phase II chemotherapy studies of the group (Jones, 1985).

3. In view of the poor prognosis, the **clinician may not wish to acknowledge this failure to the patient.** This is acceptable in that no real therapeutic alternative is presently available. At this stage in the patient's illness, i.e. with the terminal phase rapidly approaching, it may be very important for the doctor-patient relationship to be strengthened, and a suggestion to withdraw an "active" therapy could be seen as a threat to that relationship.

However, it is not so easy in practice where clear cut, black and white situations give way to a spectrum of shades of grey. It is suggested that much valuable information may be gleaned by studying this situation with a randomised trial, potentially putting an end to the uncertainty which surrounds it.

DOCUMENTATION

JONES W. J., Do we continue hormonal treatment after hormone resistance? in Therapeutic progress in Urological Cancers, pages 331-336, Murphy G. and Khoury S. editors. 1989 New York Alan R. Liss

Second Line Hormonal Treatment

S. Khoury

Urology Department, Hôpital de la Pitié, Paris, France

Not all forms of endocrine treatment produce similar results. For example, MPA compared with castration or oestrogens produced statistically lower survival rates. This highlights the fact that endocrine treatment, to produce comparable results, should reduce serum testosterone (T) to castrate levels to be at the maximum level of efficacy. This fact is confirmed by observations that bilateral orchidectomy or oestrogens only produce a second response after other first line hormonal treatments when this treatment failed to reduce T to castrate levels.

There is no good rationale to expect a second response by initiating second line endocrine treatment in patients failing control by any first line endocrine treatment with serum T levels still under castration values unless one aims to:

• *Ablate* or *block adrenal androgens*.

• See a *direct cytotoxic effect* on the tumour by using high doses of oestrogens.

• Use hormones associated with *cytotoxic drugs* such as estyracyt.

• Interfere with the production or binding of *growth factors* (Suramin).

1. Block or ablate adrenal androgens

Huggins and Scott half a century ago introduced surgical *adrenalectomy* as second line hormonal treatment. Later *hypophysectomy* was proposed, but surgical morbidity and minimal responses dampened the enthusiasm for this approach.

The introduction of drugs that inhibited adrenal steroid synthesis such as **aminoglutethimide** and high dose **ketoconazole** and, in particular, the introduction of **antiandrogens** some 20 years ago, offered a rather effective and simple means to counteract any possible stimulation of the adrenal androgens.

a) Antiandrogens

The availability and acceptable toxicity of the steroidal and non-steroidal antiandrogens with their specific ability to inhibit the binding of dihydrotestosterone (DHT) to the nuclear receptor in the prostate cancer cell, made them a popular choice to add to first line hormonal treatment in case of resistance.

Three antiandrogens are currently used (Table 1) and another, "Casodex"* is under development.

Clinical experience unfortunately does not confirm the hypothesis and objective remissions in relapsed prostate cancer by second line hormonal treatment are rare and seldom exceed 5% in most studies. However, the reported subjective remission, usually pain relief, may reach 20% of the treated

---

* "Casodex" is a trade mark, the property of Imperial Chemical Industries PLC.

Table I. Available antiandrogens commonly used in clinical treatment.

Steroidal agents
Cyproterone acetate

Non-steroidal agents
Hydroxyflutamide
Nilutamide

patients. These results, though shortlived, keep the search for active second line hormonal treatment alive.

b) Inhibitors of steroid synthesis

The blocking of the transformation of steroid precursors to steroid hormones and androgens can be achieved by aminoglutethimide and ketoconazole. Some subjective response has been seen with these drugs. Unfortunately, they inhibit the synthesis not only of androgens but also of the other steroids leading to severe complications and to the necessity for hormonal replacement therapy.

2. High doses of oestrogens

Oestrogens at high doses may have a direct cytotoxic effect on prostatic cancer cells. Some subjective (pain relief) results were recorded in hormone-refractory patients. More controlled studies are necessary to determine the exact value of this treatment.

3. Use hormones associated with cytotoxic drugs such as estracyt

Estramustine phosphate which combines chemically *oestradiol* and *nitrogen mustard,* is used in hormone-refractory patients with some objective (30%) and subjective results (40%). The mean duration of this response was 5 months.

4. Suramin

Suramin, a drug previously used for the treatment of trypanosomiasis, **blocks the binding** of several types of **growth factors**

to their corresponding cell surface receptors and is also a potent transcriptase inhibitor. These properties might explain the antiproliferative effect of this compound on cancer cells. Winnan et al. stated impressive subjective and objective responses in their patients with relapsed prostatic cancer. The experience reported by Mahler et al.was less convincing.

DOCUMENTATION

DENIS L. Current strategies in hormonal manipulation of advanced prostate cancer. Current Opinion in urology 1991, 1: 16-20.

DE VOOGT H.J. Second-line endocrine management: anti androgens and anti-oestrogens. In: Schroeder F.H., Richards B. (eds) Therapeutic Principles in Metastatic Prostate Cancer. Alan R. Liss, New York 1985: 351-357.

DROZ J.P., DE SMEDT E., KATTAN J., KEUPPENS F., KHOURY S., MAHLER C., DENIS L. Phase I- II trial with high dose fosfestrol in hormone refractory adenocarcinoma of the prostate In: Recent Advances in Urological Cancers. Diagnosis and Treatment Eds. G. Murphy, S. Khoury, C. Chatelain, L. Denis. Paris, June 27-291990: 90-91.

MAHLER C. DENIS L., DE COSTER R. The endocrine effect of ketoconazole high doses (KHD). In: Murphy GP., Khoury S., Küss R., Chatelain C., Denis L. (eds) Prostate Cancer. Part A: Research, Endocrine Treatment and Histopathology. Alan R. Liss, New York 1987:291-297.

MYERS C.E. AND LINEHAN W.M. Effect of Suramin on proliferation of human prostate carcinoma. Proc Am Assoc. Cancer Res 1989: 30:310.

IV

CHEMOTHERAPY

Chemotherapy of Prostatic Cancer : A Review

M. Robert and P., Huben

Department of Urology, Egertsville NY 14226, USA

I. INTRODUCTION

Relatively few patients are considered potential candidates for chemotherapy. Some of the reasons why chemotherapy is used only infrequently in patients with advanced, hormone refractory prostate cancer would probably include :

1) highly variable nature of prostatic cancer, from rapidly progressive to indolent and relatively asymptomatic.

2) inherent difficulties in determining response to therapy of a disease which is nonquantifiable prior to treatment and thereafter as well.

3) the advanced age, debility, and associated noncancer-related problems of the particular patient population and concern about potential toxicity.

4) reliance on hormone therapy as the endpoint of therapy.

5) the limited impact of chemotherapy to date on the progression of hormone-refractory prostate cancer.

The purpose of this chapter will be to review the clinical experience to date with chemotherapy for prostate cancer, including single-agent trials, combination therapy, and chemohormonal approaches. Because of their unquestionable significance in this area, response criteria will also be discussed.

II. RESPONSE CRITERIA

As noted, **difficulty in determining response to therapy** in patients with advanced prostate cancer has posed a critical problem in chemotherapy trials to date, and is a major cause of the wide variability of reported response rates in studies using comparable treatment regimens.

The crux of the problem is the striking but poorly understood spread of prostate cancer to bone, in which both extent of disease and therapeutic response may be evaluable but not measurable. While **bone scans** are qualitative rather than quantitative images, serial bone scans have been shown to accurately indicate the course of prostate cancer. Difficulties with the interpretation of bone scans and determining treatment response by this means have probably been overstated.

It has been suggested by others that only patients with **bidimensionally measurable soft tissue lesions** are appropriate subjects for clinical trials in which response to treatment is theend point of study. However, such rigorous evaluation requirements are unrealistic in prostate cancer patients, since only one in ten patients may be evaluable by these standards. Also, it has been suggested that patients with extensive soft tissue metastases may have a poorer survival and that these lesions are less likely to respond to chemotherapy. Response criteria should fit the disease, rather than expecting the disease to fit the response criteria.

Since *response criteria are critical factors in the study of metastatic prostate cancer, several approaches* to this problem will be discussed.

1. National Prostatic Cancer Project (NPCP) Response Criteria

A summary of NPCP response criteria is shown in Table 1. Note that all the listed criteria must be met for the response categories of *complete response*, *partial response*, and *stable disease*, while any of the listed findings would suffice for the designation of progression. Note also that both complete and partial responses require normalization of acid phosphatase, and a decrease in acid phosphatase is necessary to categorize disease as stable.

Despite the widespread application and acceptance of NPCP response criteria, criticism has centered on the significance of *"stable"* disease as a response category. It has been suggested that the stable category may include two groups of patients:

1) those who progress slowly as a function of the biology of their disease and in whom progression can only be documented over several months, and

2) patients who have an objective response to treatment and only fail to achieve a partial response by NPCP criteria because their acid phosphatase does not return all the way to normal.

In other trials in which a 50% reduction in acid phosphatase is considered significant, the NPCP "stable" patients may have been considered partial responders. Despite this problem, NPCP response criteria are still employed commonly in both the United States and Europe.

2. Eastern Cooperative Oncology Group (ECOG) Response Criteria

ECOG response criteria are summarized in Table 2. Patients are initially subdivided into those with *measurable disease* and those with *evaluable but non-measurable* disease. In those with measurable disease, complete response indicates disappearance of all measurable disease. *Partial response* indicates a 50% or greater reduction in the sum of the products of horizontal and vertical tumor diameters. No change indicates an increase of less than 25% of the products, while progression indicates an increase of more than 25%.

The endpoint of drug assessment in patients with evaluable but non-measurable disease is *survival time*, and certain indicators of response are used as guidelines for continuing or discontinuing chemotherapy. All patients in this group require a minimum of six weeks of treatment to be evaluable. Indicators for continuation of treatment include performance status, pain score, and body weight. Patients in whom performance status has worsened one or more levels at 6 weeks discontinue initial treatment, while patients must show an improvement of at least one level at 12 weeks to continue initial treatment. Pain must be moderate or severe to be evaluable, with interval trends similar to those of performance status for continuation of therapy. If patients lose more than 5 % of dry body weight during the first 12 weeks of treatment, they cross over to Phase II arms or go off study.

3. European Organization for Research on Treatment of Cancer (EORTC) Response Criteria

EORTC response criteria, as they apply to metastatic prostate cancer, are summarized in Table 3. *Subcategories* in this classification include *objective specific* criteria, *objective nonspecific* criteria, and *subjective* criteria. *Objective specific criteria*

TABLE 1. NPCP response criteria

Indicator	Complete response	Partial response	Stable response	Progression
	ALL:	ALL:	ALL:	ANY:
Tumor masses	disappear	1 ↓ by > 50 %	none ↑ > 25 %	> 25 % ↑
New lesions	none	none	none	yes
Elevated acid phos.	normalizes	normalizes	↓	same/ ↑
Bone scan	normalizes	improved	stable	↑
Osteolytic lesions	all recalcify	some recalcify	stable	↑
Osteoblastic lesions	normalize	stabilize	stable	↑
Hepatomegaly	normalizes	at least 30 % ↓	< 30 % ↑	↑
Performance status	stable	stable	stable	↑ anemia

TABLE 2. ECOG response criteria

Indicator	Complete response	Partial response	No change	Progression
a) *Measurable:*				
new lesions	none	none	none	yes
sum of products of ←↑↓→ tumor diameters	complete disappearance	⩾ 50 % ↓	< 25 % ↑	> 25 % ↑
liver enlargement	normalizes	> 30 % ↓	< 25 % ↑	> 25 % ↑
lytic bone lesions	normalizes	50 % ↓	< 50 % ↓	> 25 % ↑
acid phosphatase	normalizes	> 50 % ↓	< 50 % ↓	> 50 % ↑
b) *Non-measurable:* survival time				

TABLE 3. EORTC response criteria

Indicator	Objective regression	Status quo	Failure
a) *bone metastases only*			
new lesions	none	none	yes
blastic lesions	stable or 1 ↓	stable	↑
lytic lesions	↓ of ½	↓ of < ½	↑
acid phosphatase	↓ ⩾ 50 %	< 50 % ↓	↑
alkaline phosphatase	↓	stable	↑
prostate primary	↓ /stable	stable	↑
b) *bone and/or visceral metastases*	as above, *or:*		
measurable lesions	↓ of ⩾ ½, if ⩾ 4	< ½ ↓	↑

TABLE 4. Summary of NPCP single agent trials in patients with hormone-refractory prostate cancer and *without* prior radiation therapy

Protocol	Agent	CR/PR	Stable	Response rate	Progression
100	Cyclophosphamide	7 %	39 %	46 %	54 %
	5-Fluorouracil	12 %	24 %	36 %	64 %
	Standard therapy	0	19 %	19 %	81 %
300	Cyclophosphamide	0	26 %	26 %	74 %
	DTIC	4 %	23 %	27 %	73 %
	Procarbazine	0	14 %	14 %	86 %
700	Cyclophosphamide	7 %	28 %	35 %	65 %
	Hydroxyurea	8 %	7 %	15 %	85 %
	Methyl-CCNU	4 %	26 %	30 %	70 %
1100	Methotrexate	5 %	36 %	41 %	59 %
	Cisplatinum	4 %	32 %	36 %	64 %
	Estramustine	2 %	32 %	34 %	66 %

apply to the prostate primary, cutaneous lesions or superficial lymph nodes, bone lesions, distant visceral lesions, and acid phosphatase level. Objective regression occurs in bone metastases when lytic lesions recalcify or when no new abnormal bone formation occurs in blastic lesions and the bone scan does not worsen. A 50% decrease in an elevated acid phosphatase level during therapy is considered one of the criteria of objective specific improvement. **Objective nonspecific criteria** include upper urinary tract dilatation, neurologic findings, alkaline phosphatase levels, and ambulatory status. These criteria must be unchanged or improved in the case of objective regression. Pain is the only subjective criterion.

When evaluable disease is **bone metastases** only, the criteria of objective regression are disappearance of at least one blastic lesion or no further calcium deposits on bone X-rays, a decrease in serum acid phosphatase of at least 50%, and regression of the primary tumor. In patients with both bone and visceral metastases, the same criteria as above would indicate objective regression. When bone lesions are unchanged in this situation, then there must be measurable regression of at least one-half on the distant or visceral metastases, provided that there are at least 4 measurable lesions.

As a brief review of the above response criteria indicates, determination of treatment response in metastatic prostate cancer is highly variable, arbitrary, and complicated. It is probable that future indicators of response will involve analysis of survival or progression-free survival. This approach has its own problems, since recognized prognostic indicators such as performance status, pain status, previous response to hormone therapy, and age at diagnosis will have a significant impact on survival data (13). The potential role of prostate specific antigen or PSA as a response indicator is largely undetermined. It is clear, however, that response rates and survival data are largely meaningless outside the context of large, randomized, and controlled clinical studies, in which the impact of both patient and disease variability will be lessened.

III. SINGLE AGENT TRIALS

The results of single-agent chemotherapy trials for advanced prostate cancer have been the topic of numerous reviews. The largest series of single-agent chemotherapy

TABLE 5. Summary of NPCP single agent trials in patients with hormone-refractory prostate cancer and *with* prior radiation therapy

Protocol	Agent	CR/PR	Stable	Response rate	Progression
200	Estramustine	6 %	24 %	30 %	70 %
	Streptozoticin	0	32 %	32 %	68 %
	Standard Therapy	0	19 %	19 %	81 %
400	Prednimustine	0	13 %	13 %	87 %
	Prednimustine + Estramustine	2 %	11 %	13 %	87 %
800	Estramustine	4 %	22 %	26 %	74 %
	Vincristine	3 %	12 %	15 %	85 %
	Vincristine + Estramustine	0	24 %	24 %	76 %
1200	Estramustine	0	18 %	18 %	82 %
	Cis-platinum	0	21 %	21 %	79 %
	Cis-platinum + Estramustine	0	33 %	33 %	67 %

TABLE 6. Combinaison chemotherapy trials

Author	Agents	No. pts.	Objective response rate	Response criteria
Ihde, et al. (1980)	Doxorubicin Cyclophosphamide	32	7 (22 %)	——
Herr (1982)	Methotrexate 5-fluorouracil Cyclophosphamide	20	3 (15 %)	NPCP
Stephens, et al. (1984)	Doxorubicin Cyclophosphamide	19	6 (32 %)	SWOG
Babaian, Hsu (1984)	5-fluorouracil doxorubicin Mitomycin-C (FAM)	14	0	NPCP
Page, et al. (1985)	Doxorubicin Lomustine	22	12 (57 %)	NPCP
	Cyclophosphamide 5-fluorouracil	25	2 (8 %)	NPCP
Logothetis, et al. (1983)	Doxorubicin mitomycin-C 5-fluorouracil (DMF)	62	30 (48 %)	——
Burk, et al. (1987)	Doxorubicin mitomycin-C 5-fluorouracil (DMF)	86	22 (26 %)	NPCP
Droz, et al. (1987)	Doxorubicin 5-fluorouracil Cis-platinum (FAP)	15	2 (13 %)	NPCP

trials has been that of the National Prostatic Cancer Project (17). Results of the trials conducted by the NPCP are shown in Tables 4 and 5.

IV. COMBINATION CHEMOTHERAPY TRIALS

The results of several representative trials of combination chemotherapy are shown in Table 6. While the results of these trials seem encouraging, most reviewers have stated that there is little if any evidence that combination therapy is more effective than single agent chemotherapy. While testis and bladder cancer chemotherapy clearly illustrate the additive or synergistic effects of combination therapy, this has not been demonstrated in the case of prostate cancer.

In fact, *the potential benefit of chemotherapy for prostate cancer has been questioned*. Eisenberger and associates have stated that "the palliative role of nonhormonal cytotoxic chemotherapy in the treatment of endocrine-resistant prostate carcinoma has not been established". In this review, they stated that only about 5% of patients demonstrate the criteria of **partial** or **complete response** to chemotherapy. The authors felt that **stable disease** is a **questionable indicator** of treatment response and that better indicators are needed for both treatment response and quality of life determinations. They concluded that **survival** should be a major endpoint of response in future trials and that such trials should include a control arm of best symptomatic care or second-line endocrine therapy. While most of these conclusions are quite constructive, it can only be hoped that the impact of this report will not dampen enthusiasm for or interest in further clinical studies of prostate cancer chemotherapy.

V. CHEMOHORMONAL TRIALS

1. NPCP trials

There were 3 NPCP trials conducted which compared hormone therapy alone to chemotherapy plus hormone therapy in patients with **newly diagnosed** metastatic prostate cancer.

The first was NPCP Protocol 500, in which previously untreated patients were randomized to one of the following arms : 1) DES 1 mg orally 3 times a day, or orchiectomy ; 2) DES plus cyclophosphamide at mg/m² IV every 3 weeks ; or 3) estramustine phosphate at 600 mg/m² orally daily plus cyclophosphamide. In 246 evaluable patients, initial objective response rates at 12 weeks were not significantly different. There was a slight improvement in survival in patients on the chemotherapy arms, particularly in patients with pain at presentation. Chemotherapy toxicity was not excessive.

The second NPCP study of **hormone therapy** versus **hormone therapy plus chemotherapy** versus **chemohormonal therapy** was Protocol 1300, in which a total of 296 evaluable patients were randomized to one of 3 treatment arms : 1) DES or orchiectomy; 2) estramustine phosphate 600 mg/m² daily; or 3) cyclophosphamide 1mg/m² IV weekly. In this study, there were non significant differences in the distribution of objective, short-term responses or in overall survival. Hematologic toxicity was significantly higher in the combination chemotherapy group.

The third and final NPCP study comparing **hormone therapy** to **hormone therapy plus chemotherapy** in patients with newly diagnosed metastatic prostate cancer was Protocol 1700, the results of which were recently reported. A total of 265 patients were randomized to one of 3 treatment arms : 1) DES or orchiectomy ; 2) the luteinizing hormone-releasing hormone (LHRH) analog buserelin ; or 3) methotrexate 40 mg/m², then 60 mg on day 8 and every 14 days thereafter, plus DES or orchiectomy. In 261 evaluable patients, there was no significant difference in survival among the 3 groups.

2. Androgen priming and chemotherapy

The results of a multicenter randomized clinical trial examining the role of androgen priming and chemotherapy in patients with **hormone refractory metastatic prostate cancer** have recently been reported (24). All of 85 men were treated continuously with aminoglutethimide and hydrocortisone to suppress adrenal androgen secretion and received cyclic intravenous chemotherapy. Aminoglutethimide was given at a dose of 250 mg orally twice a day, then increased to 250 mg 4 times a day after 2 weeks. A total of 40 mg of hydrocortisone was given orally daily in 3 divided doses. Chemotherapy consisted initially of cyclophosphamide 500 mg/m², 5-fluorouracil 500 mg/m², and doxorubicin 50 mg/m² every 3 weeks until a maximum cumulative dosage of 400 mg/m² of doxorubicin was reached. Thereafter, chemotherapy was changed to high-dose methotrexate at 200 mg/m², then 5-fluorouracil 600 mg/m², followed by leucovorin rescue 24 hours later at 10 mg/m² 4 times a day for 6 doses, given every 4 weeks. Patients randomized to the androgen stimulation arm received the synthetic androgen fluoxymestrone 5 mg orally twice a day for 3 days before and on the day of chemotherapy administration. The *ratio-nale* for this approach is the assumption that androgens stimulate prostate cancer growth and that *chemotherapy is more effective against rapidly proliferating cells*. NPCP response criteria were used, with the exception that a 50% decrease (rather than normalization) of acid phosphatase was considered to be indicative of an objective response.

In 61 evaluable patients, response rate (remission plus stabilization) was not significantly different between the stimulation (79%) and control (73%) arms. Median duration of response was also similar for the stimulation (9 months) and control (10 months) arms. There was a statistically significant difference in median survival between the two groups, with better survival in the control group (15 months) compared to the stimulation group (10 months). Spinal cord compression developed in 2 patients during the first cycle of androgen priming and chemotherapy, which prompted the authors to perform a screening myelogram in all patients randomized to the stimulation arm. However, 2 patients in the control arm also developed cord compression. Most patients experienced worsening bone pain during androgen priming, which usually lessened considerably after a few cycles of therapy. While the authors concede that it is impossible to determine from this study

which treatment component (androgen ablation or chemotherapy) was more beneficial, they concluded that androgen priming does not enhance the efficacy of cytotoxic chemotherapy but is actually associated with a worse outcome.

While the results of other studies employing androgen priming to enhance chemotherapeutic effect have been largely inconclusive, this and other studies strongly suggest that androgen priming must be applied with extreme caution in this patient population.

VI. CONCLUSION

The many problems and controversies which become apparent in discussing the role of chemotherapy for metastatic prostate cancer underscore the need for renewed interest in this area. While it is easy to criticize many of the studies to date, they represent the beginning of a systematic approach to the problems. The definition and standardization of response criteria remains a critical issue. Multi-institutional and cooperative groups, both in the United States and abroad, should take a leading role in addressing this problem and the direction of future clinical trials. If one considers the potential impact worldwide of an effective treatment for hormone-refractory, metastatic prostate cancer, the need to pursue further scientific and clinical studies in this field is apparent.

DOCUMENTATION

CHISHOLM GD, STONE AR, BEYNON LI, MERRICK MV. The bone scan as a tumor marker in prostatic carcinoma. Eur. Urol. 8 : 257-260, 1982.

GIBBONS RP. Prostate Cancer Chemotherapy. CANCER 60 : 586-588, 1987.

HUBEN RP, MURPHY GP, and the Investigators of the National Prostatic Cancer Project. A comparison of diethylstilbestrol or orchiectomy with buserelin and with methotrexate plus diethylstilbestrol or orchiectomy in newly diagnosed patients with clinical Stage D2 cancer of the prostate. Cancer 62 : 1881-1887, 1988.

INDICATIONS

I

STAGE T1 (A)

Management of Stage A (T1) Prostate Cancer

Joseph A. Smith, Jr, Yong-Hyun Cho,
Division of Urology, University of Utah, Salt Lake City, Utah, USA

I. INCIDENCE AND DEFINITION

According to the American College of Surgeons survey, 26% of patients with adenocarcinoma of the prostate present with stage T1 disease. By definition, such tumours are nonpalpable.

Historically, the diagnosis has been established almost routinely as an **incidental finding** in patients undergoing transurethral prostatectomy for bladder outlet obstruction by presumed benign prostatic hyperplasia (10% of the cases).

Increasingly, though, transrectal ultrasonography and prostate-specific antigen levels are identifying patients with nonpalpable prostate tumours.

Non palpable tumours encompass a spectrum extending from prostatic intraepithelial neoplasia (PIN) to diffuse high-grade tumours. A meaningful subclassification should separate patients with biologically insignificant disease from those whose tumours seem destined to cause morbidity or even death.

Undoubtedly, some patients with stage T1 prostate cancer suffer disease progression and tumour-related death. However, the majority of patients have tumour that is likely to remain clinically insignificant during their lifetimes. This is the basis for the attempts at substaging of stage T1 in to stage T1a (A1), presumedly associated with low morbidity and mortality and stage T1b (A2), presumedly biologically more active. This is a fundamental issue which has profound implications for the management of stage T1 prostate cancer.

A rational treatment policy should be based on an attempt to *spare morbidity for the substantial majority of patients not in need of therapy while selectively applying definitive treatment to those with clinically significant disease.*

The main **criteria** used commonly to subclassify T1 into T1a and Tlb are the **tumour volume** and tumour **grade** in the resected specimen.

In practice there are some difficulties in establishing such classification and its clinical significance.

1. Tumour volume.

At the present time, there is no uniform agreement in the literature about the appropriate **volume measurements** to distinguish T1a from T1b cancer.

Simple **counting of the chips** is used in some series, with fewer than three or five chips involved with cancer being considered stage T1a tumour.

More commonly, the total involvement of the specimen with tumour is estimated, with 5% or less being considered stage T1a disease.

Tumour volume at the time of detection is a powerful prognostic indicator. Stamey and associates have shown that virtually all cancers with a volume of more than 3 cc have extraprostatic extension, whereas those of less than 1 cc usually are confined within the prostatic capsule.

Several problems arise in using these data to make clinical decisions about patients with nonpalpable prostate cancer, however.

a) Determination of tumour volume by any method, including transrectal ultrasonography, is **notoriously inaccurate**, often underestimating the volume of tumour

b) Although small volume tumours frequently are confined within the prostatic capsule, there is **no method for identifying those tumours destined to grow** and become clinically significant in the patient's lifetime.

There is no evidence that continued monitoring of patients by digital rectal examination, transrectal ultrasonography, prostate-specific antigen levels, or combinations of the above will identify growth of the tumour at a point when intervention still may be curative.

c) How should nonpalpable tumours detected by ultrasonography be classified? Newer staging systems address this issue, but uncertainties regarding the natural history of such disease and the prognosis for small nonpalpable tumours confound the problem.

2. Grade

Any high-grade lesion (Gleason sum of 7 or higher) is considered to be stage T1b disease. In fact, few patients with volume criteria for T1a cancer actually have high-grade tumours causing a reclassification as stage T1b.

Tumour grade is a powerful prognostic indicator for all stages of prostate cancer. Although exceptions abound, low-grade or well-differentiated tumours generally carry a better prognosis than high-grade, poorly differentiated lesions.

Unfortunately, tumour grade often is not helpful in small nonpalpable prostate cancers. Most often, low-volume tumours are of low grade. Furthermore, **flow cytometry** frequently does not provide unique information, because a diploid histogram usually is seen in small tumours. Thus, a key issue remains a dilemma. **Presumably, even tumours destined to attain large size and metastasize are of low volume at some time in their natural history**. Nevertheless, high-grade malignant cells or an aneuploid cell population are rarely identified in small-volume tumours.

II. HOW DO WE DETECT NONPALPABLE TUMOURS OF THE PROSTATE

1. TURP

Nonpalpable tumours of the prostate are mainly detected as an incidental finding in patients undergoing transurethral prostatectomy for bladder outlet obstruction by presumed benign prostatic hyperplasia.

2. Non palpable tumours are increasingly detected before TUR by transrectal ultrasonography, biopsy and prostate-specific antigen levels

a. TRUS

The peripheral zone of the gland is the origin for almost 80 per cent of prostatic adenocarcinomas. Although ultrasonography is able to detect some small peripheral tumours that are not palpable, most peripheral zone tumours are accessible for digital palpation. Nearly 20 per cent of prostate adenocarcinomas arise from the transition zone. This probably includes the majority of nonpalpable tumours and those that classically comprise stage T1 disease. Because the transition zone surrounds the urethra and is the origin of BPH, it is primarily transition zone tissue that is removed during a transurethral resection of the prostate. Although transrectal ultrasonography is an accurate method for identifying tumours in the peripheral zone, it is less reliable for the detection of transition zone cancers.

b) Biopsy

Agatstein et al performed blind needle aspiration biopsies of the prostate in 102 men undergoing transurethral prostatectomy. Fifteen patients had stage T1a tumours, but none was identified preoperatively. Four patients had stage T1b disease, and cytology showed malignant cells in three.

c) PSA

Prostate-specific antigen levels may be elevated in patients with nonpalpable cancer, but most patients with stage T1 adenocarcinoma of the prostate do not have elevated prostate specific antigen. In addition, these patients have benign prostatic hyperplasia, which may contribute to the serum prostatespecific antigen level before transurethral resection of the prostate. Prostate-specific antigen levels should fall after transurethral prostatectomy. A "normal" value after transurethral resection of the prostate has not been established. Nevertheless, a rising prostate specific antigen concentration after transurethral prostatectomy may indicate tumour progression and should lead to prostate biopsies to detect residual carcinoma.

Overall, there currently is no reliable method for the detection of transition zone or stage T1 cancers prior to transurethral prostatectomy. A low rate of detection occurs with blind biopsies, and neither transrectal ultrasound nor prostate-specific antigen provides sufflcient sensitivity or specificity in the detection of stage T1 carcinoma.

Therefore, for most patients with no palpable abnormalities of the prostate suggestive of carcinoma, transurethral prostatectomy can be performed without further efforts to detect stage T1 carcinoma preoperatively.

III. NATURAL HISTORY OF STAGE T1 CARCINOMA

The most important factor influencing the management of stage T1 carcinoma of the prostate is the predicted natural history of untreated disease.

1. Natural history as predicted by the data from the first TURP:

The information gathered at the time of the first TURP are the basis for the substaging between T1a and T1b, as discussed above, and this subclassification has been extensively used in an attempt to predict the natural history of non palpable prostate cancers.

a) Stage T1b:

Although there is little information available about the natural history of untreated stage T1b carcinoma, a relatively poor prognosis if left untreated is implied by several findings.

• Some 25% of patients undergoing pelvic lymph node dissection for clinical stage T1b carcinoma of the prostate are found to have *histologic evidence of nodal metastasis.*

• In patients with stage T1b tumours who undergo radical prostatectomy, the significant majority are found to have *residual cancer* present within the prostate. The tumour diffusely involves the prostate in most of these patients (Table 1). Paulson and coworkers performed radical prostatectomy in 69 patients with stage T1b carcinoma. Thirty-four patients (49%) had tumour that was not considered organ confined. Twenty-four patients (35%) had margin-positive radical prostatectomy specimens, and 17 (25%) had seminal vesicle involvement.

• In sum, stage T1b carcinoma is a clinically significant disease in most patients.

b) Stage T1a

In contrast, there are several studies suggesting a *low rate of progressive disease* and an even lower rate of death from carcinoma of the prostate in stage T1a disease.

• Cantrell and associates originally published data showing only a 2% progression rate for stage T1a carcinoma. In a follow-up to this study, it was reported that *16% of patients at risk for 8 years or longer had disease progression.* However, almost half of the patients were excluded from analysis because they died from other causes within 8 years or had not been followed for a full 8 years. Censoring of patients because of death from other causes seems to eliminate the consideration that one of the reasons that stage T1a disease is clinically insignificant in most patients is that there is a high incidence of competing causes of death in elderly men. Furthermore, this study examined only the rate of progressive disease, *which does not necessarily equate with death from prostate cancer.*

• Lowe and colleagues retrospectively analyzed patients with stage T1a disease and found that *9% suffered progression* with a median follow-up of 9 years using tumour extent alone as a criterion for stage T1a.

However, *death* from prostate cancer occurred in only *1% of these patients*.

• Hanash and coworkers reported that untreated patients with stage T1a prostate cancer had a life expectancy similar to that of age-matched controls.

• Somewhat *in contrast to these studies,* Blute and associates found disease progression in *24% of patients aged 60 or younger at the time of diagnosis.* This is a very interesting study regardig the potential morbidity of stage T1a prostate cancer, as it stresses a very noteworthy point: *because young patients may be at risk for many years, the disease progression rate in this group justifies greater concern.* Our understanding and management of stage T1a disease ought to take very much into account the age of the patient.

2. The role of repeat TURP

On the assumption that transurethral prostatectomy may only have sampled the lesion, leaving behind undetected diffuse carcinoma, TURP has been advocated as a method to detect residual cancer left behind after the first TURP.

▪ At the University of Utah, we have performed a repeat resection in 55 patients with stage T1a adenocarcinoma. No further tumour was found in 45 (82%), whereas isolated foci of cancer were found in 8 patients (14%) (see Table 1). We made the decision that none of these patients should be reclassified as having stage T1b disease. Two

Table 1. Pathologic findings on repeat transurethral resection or radical prostatectomy in stage T1 carcinoma.

PROCEDURE (NO. OF PATIENTS)	NO. WITHOUT RESIDUAL TUMOR (%)	NO. WITH RESIDUAL TUMOR, FOCAL (%)	NO. WITH RESIDUAL TUMOR, DIFFUSE (%)
Repeat TUR (55)	45 (82)	9 (14.5)	2 (3.5)
Radical prostatectomy (31)	16 (52)	11 (35)	4 (13)
TOTAL (86)	61 (71)	19 (22)	6 (7)

From Smith JA Jr: Stage A carcinoma of the prostate. *In* Smith JA Jr, Middleton RG (eds): Clinical Management of Prostate Cancer. Chicago, Year Book Medical Publishers, 1987, p 90; with permission.

patients (4%) did have diffuse foci of carcinoma detected, and the disease was reclassified as stage T1b. On the basis of this series, it was concluded at the University of Utah, that repeat transurethral resection was not a useful procedure in most patients. The histologic findings on the original resected tissue appear to reflect disease status accurately in the substantial majority of patients.

3. Natural history of nonpalpable tumours detected by ultrasonography and biopsy.

It is even more difficult to make statements regarding the clinical and biologic significance of nonpalpable tumours detected by methods other than transurethral prostatectomy.

a) Tumours discovered by ultrasonography

Stamey and associates have shown that tumour volume correlates closely with local disease stage: patients with a tumour volume of greater than 3 cc frequently have extracapsular extension, whereas lesions smaller than 1 cc usually are organ confined. Although these data can be used to predict local tumour extent and, implicitly, prognosis at a defined point in time, they do not allow identification of patients with low-volume disease who are destined to have rapid tumour growth and disease-related morbidity if left untreated.

b) Tumours discovered by biopsy

As transrectal ultrasound is an inaccurate method for determining the volume of transition zone tumours, it has been suggested that volume calculations can be based on the amount of tumour present in core biopsy specimens. *Tumour that extends for less than 2 mm along a core biopsy may be considered clinically and biologically insignificant* by these calculations. Careful follow-up using digital rectal examination,

transrectal ultrasound, and prostate-specific antigen has been recommended as a method for monitoring disease in these patients.

In conclusion, there are no longitudinal survival data available on which to base recommendations for the management of patients with nonpalpable prostate cancer detected by needle biopsy rather than transurethral prostatectomy. However, it seems logical to conclude that many of these patients have biologically insignificant disease that does not warrant definitive therapy. The presence of **high grade** cancer, an ultrasonographically measured tumour of **greater than 1 cc** in volume, or **diffuse** carcinoma on multiple biopsies **probably justifies aggressive treatment**. For incidentally discovered carcinoma that is apparently both low volume and low grade, there are no data confirming the hypothesis that careful follow-up surveillance by any method will accurately allow identification of tumour progression, but this seems to be a rational approach for most such patients.

IV. RESULTS OF DEFINITIVE THERAPY

As with other stages of apparently localized prostate cancer, the primary treatment options for stage T1 carcinoma are radical prostatectomy and external-beam irradiation. Typically, variations in patient selection, staging, treatment method, and duration of follow-up vary, making comparison of different series difflcult.

1. Radical Prostatectomy

a) Stage T1a

A group of patients with stage T1a carcinoma of the prostat underwent pelvic lymph node dissection and radical prostatectomy at the University of Utah. Although we no longer consider it appropriate therapy at our hospital for most patients with stage T1a tumours, interesting and relevant data can be obtained from examination of this series.

Forty-one patients underwent pelvic lymph node dissection as a staging procedure for T1a carcinoma. None of these patients had pelvic lymph node metastases identified histologically. Sixteen of thirty-one patients (51%) had no residual foci of carcinoma identified, whereas 11 (36%) had isolated foci of well-differentiated carcinoma, and 4 patients (13%) had diffuse residual carcinoma.

Histologic data cannot necessarily be used to predict tumour behaviour. Nevertheless, because there is a correlation between tumour volume and prognosis, some extrapolation of these data is valid. Detection of residual carcinoma does not necessarily imply that the radical prostatectomy was justified, because occasional foci of well-differentiated carcinoma rarely mean progression to clinically significant disease or cancer-related death. Thus, few patients with isolated foci of well differentiated carcinoma on a transurethral resection specimen have anything more than further isolated well-differentiated foci at radical prostatectomy. Rarely, then, is significant residual disease left behind after a transurethral specimen shows T1a carcinoma.

b) Stage T1b:

The differing prognosis for stage T1b cancer compared with stage T1a is reflected in the results and findings after radical prostatectomy. 24% of patients with clinical stage T1b carcinoma on whom we have performed pelvic lymph node dissection have had histologic metastatic disease. This figure is consistent with the findings from other studies.

It is unusual for the radical prostatectomy specimen of patients with stage T1b tumours not to show at least some carcinoma, and the tumour is usually diffuse (Table 2). Significantly, Paulson and coworkers found seminal vesicle invasion in 25% of their patients with stage T1b disease undergoing radical prostatectomy, and 49% had tumour that was not organ confined.

These figures are similar to those seen with clinical stage T2c lesions but also are somewhat higher than in comparable series of stage T1b patients.

Survival data after radical prostatectomy seem to justify the procedure in patients with T1b carcinoma. In our series, 65% of the patients are alive and free of disease 10 years after radical prostatectomy, and cancer death has occurred in only 10 per cent. *These results appear to be significantly better than those obtained with expectant management alone.*

2. External Irradiation

There are few studies reporting a minimum of a 10-year follow-up of patients with stage T1b prostate cancer treated by irradiation. Also, in many series, adequate staging of

Table 2. Pathologic findings from radical prostatectomy and pelvic lymphadenectomy according to Grade in patients with stage T1b carcinoma.

NO. OF PTS.	GLEASON SCORE	NO. WITH RESIDUAL TUMOR			
		None (%)	Focal (%)	Diffuse (%)	Pos. Nodes (%)
11	2–4	3 (27)	3 (27)	5 (46)	0
5	5–7	0	2 (13.5)	11 (73)	2 (13.5)
8	8–10	0	1 (12.5)	7 (88)	6 (75)

From Smith JA Jr: Stage A carcinoma of the prostate. *In* Smith JA Jr, Middleton RG (eds): Clinical Management of Prostate Cancer. Chicago, Year Book Medical Publishers, 1987, p 90; with permission.

the pelvic lymph nodes was not performed, which may adversely affect the results, as patients with positive nodes usually are excluded from radical prostatectomy series. The methods for lymph node evaluation vary in different series. Because pelvic lymph node metastasis is rare in patients with stage T1a lesions, lymph node evaluation is not warranted. Pelvic node metastasis is found by CT scanning or lymphangiography in fewer than 10 per cent of patients with stage T1b carcinoma, significantly less than the 25 per cent incidence found by pelvic lymph node dissection. On the other hand, reported series of stage T1 carcinoma treated by irradiation often categorize T1a and T1b disease together, which would have a significantly favorable impact on the results.

The series of Bagshaw and associates historically have included stage T1 cancers in the category of "disease limited to the prostate," which also includes stage T2 cancers. In a recent updated review published in this book patients are segregated into T1a and T1b categories. Surprisingly, little difference in survival is noted between these groups.

McGowan reported a 97 per cent 5-year survival rate in patients with stage T1 carcinoma treated by external-beam irradiation. This series included a significant number of patients with stage T1a tumours, and follow-up of 5 years clearly is insufficient to justify any comment regarding treatment efficacy.

V. SUMMARY AND RECOMMENDATIONS

Stage T1 carcinoma of the prostate historically encompasses disease causing *no palpable abnormality* of the prostate that is discovered incidentally after a transurethral prostatectomy.

Transrectal ultrasonography has defined a new group of patients with nonpalpable tumours *diagnosed by needle biopsy*. How these two groups of patients interrelate remains unclear, and new issues regarding the biologic significance of low volume disease have emerged.

It is important and pertinent to *understand exactly what has occurred when a transurethral resection for presumed benign prostatic hyperplasia shows adenocarcinoma* on histologic examination. At autopsy, almost *30% of men over the age of 65 will have microscopic evidence of adenocarcinoma* of the prostate if careful examination is performed. However, screening studies using ultrasonography with multiple biopsies or a rectal examination detect cancer in fewer than 5% of men. Moreover, only a small overall percentage of men with prostate cancer are destined to die from their disease.

A transurethral resection of the prostate is merely an extended sampling of tissue which, by virtue of the figures cited above, is likely to discover incidental cancer in some patients. The sheer weight of numbers suggests that the *overwhelming majority of these patients will not die from cancer* of the prostate even in the absence of any treatment.

Treatment of any disease requires an informed and judicious application of certain principles. The natural history of the disease, as well as the results and morbidity of therapy, must be considered. Finally, selective application of treatment to patients most likely to benefit should be employed.

1. Stage T1a

Stage T1a carcinoma of the prostate progresses to clinically significant disease in a distinct minority of patients. Even in this group, the median time to progression is protracted, and progression does not necessarily equate with significant morbidity or death from the disease.

Although the technique for radical prostatectomy has improved in recent years, it is still a major surgical procedure with attendant morbidity.

For the typical patient with stage T1a carcinoma of the prostate, the *risk of death from prostate cancer does not justify an aggressive approach* : neither external irradiation nor radical prostatectomy is appropriate. Disease status should be monitored with periodic rectal examination, prostate-specific antigen assay, and transrectal ultrasonography. Although this approach seems logical, it is unproved whether the use of prostate-specific antigen and transrectal ultrasound in the follow-up of these patients will allow more accurate and early detection of disease progression.

There is, however, a growing concern that, in *young patients, even a stage T1a tumour might progress to become clinically meaningful,* which would indicate serious consideration to radical modalities of treatment in some of these younger patients.

2. Stage T1b

The incidence of pelvic lymph node metastasis, the volume of residual tumour, the histologic findings at radical prostatectomy, and the longitudinal follow-up of patients combine to support the belief that stage T1b carcinoma *is a virulent disease* in most patients. *Aggressive therapy with curative intent thus is justified in patients of appropriate age and health*. Both radical prostatectomy and external irradiation appear to provide long-term survival rates superior to those obtained by observation alone, although nearly 20% of patients die from carcinoma despite therapy.

Is there a reliable method to determine the prognosis in an individual patient ?

Unfortunately, *there is no reliable method* to determine the prognosis in an individual patient or to distinguish the small number of patients with incidentally discovered, nonpalpable prostate cancer who are destined to develop disease progression and die from the majority who have biologically and clinically insignificant disease. Emerging recommendations that *careful surveillance* be employed in some of these patients seem valid and logical, *but the success of such a policy in identifying disease progression at a point when intervention is still potentially curative has not been demonstrated*. Efforts to identify individual prognostic features must continue.

In the meantime, emotional arguments that all cancer must be treated when discovered should be suppressed by an informed and objective understanding of the natural history of nonpalpable prostate cancer and the potential impact of treatment.

DOCUMENTATION

BLUTE ML, ZINCKE H, FARROW GM: Long-term follow-up of young patients with stage A adenocarcinoma of the prostate. J Urol 136:840-843, 1986.

EPSTEIN JI, WALSH PC, EGGLESTON JC: Prognosis of untreated stage A1 prostate carcinoma: A study of 94 cases with extended follow-up abstract. J Urol 135:242A, 1986.

LOWE BA, LISTROM MB: Incidental carcinoma of the prostate: An analysis of the predictors of progression. J Urol 140:1340-1344, 1988.

PAULSON DF, STONE AR, WALTHER PJ, et al: Radical prostatectomy: Anatomic predictors of success or failure. J Urol 136:1041-1044, 1986.

SMITH JA Jr: Stage A carcinoma of the prostate. In Clinical Management of Prostatic Cancer. Chicago, Year Book Medical Publishers, pp 85-96, 1988.

SMITH JA JR, GLEIDMAN JA, MIDDLETON RG: Pelvic lymph node metastasis from prostate cancer: Influence of tumour grade and stage in 452 consecutive patients. J Urol 130:290-292,1983.

The predictive significance of substaging stage T1 (A) prostate cancer (T1a versus T1b) for volume and grade of total cancer in the prostate.

Gunther E. Voges, John McNeal, Elsie A. Redwine, Fuad S. Freiha and Thomas Stamey.

Division of Urology, Stanford University School of Medicine, Stanford, California.

J. Urol., 147, 858, 1992

Recently, **doubts have been raised about the consistently benign course of stage T1 (A) cancer of the prostate.**

In this study, we did a morphometric analysis on 44 radical prostatectomy specimens for 22 clinical stage T1a and 22 clinical stage T1b *to assess the value of the T1a/T1b subclassification to predict the residual volume of cancer within the prostate (hence, the total volume of cancer, which seems a key indicator of future biological behavior).*

I. MATERIAL AND METHOD

All radical prostatectomy specimens were processed by the Stanford technique as described previously.

Cancer volume was calculated as the sum of tumor areas measured by computer from the tracing of the slides, multiplied by the section thickness, and multiplied by a factor of 1.5 to correct for tissue shrinkage during processing.

The volume of the resected cancer (TUR) and the volume of residual cancer (radical prostatectomy) were added to give the **total volume** of stage T1 cancer.

Estimating that the smallest detectable (by DRE) cancers of clinical importance have a volume of about 0.2 cc, **any cancer 0.2 cc or more was considered significant.**

II. RESULTS.

1. Morphology of stage T1 carcinoma:

Total volumes ranged from 0.03 to 11.3 cc, median 0.63 cc (Figure 1).

Residual cancer was found in 44 cases (95.4%), its volume **greater than 1cc in 11 stage T1a and 14 stage T1b cancers.**

In **6 cases no residual resection cancer** was found in the radical prostatectomy specimen (4 stage T1a and 2 stage T1b).

Although it has been estimated that 25% of all prostate cancer arise in the transition zone, 86% of the cancers in this series were transition zone cancers.

Five of the 6 non transition zone cancers in this series were all peripheral zone cancers, ranging in volume from 1.4 to 8.3 cc.

2. Clinical substaging (T1a / T1b) versus total cancer volume and grade:

A cutoff volume of 1 cc gave the best separation betwen stage T1a and stage T1b. There were 6 stage T1a larger than 1 cc and 4 stage T1b smaller than 1 cc. **Thus, 23% of the cases were misclassified** (Figure 1).

Using only residual cancer volume with a threshold of 0.6 cc, 6 stage T1a exceeded the threshold and 8 stage T1b were below it, yelding a 32% misclassification rate.

Grade 4 or more was a more reliable index of large volume cancers than percent of tumor in the TURP, although **8 cancers were undergraded based on the resection specimen alone.**

3. Residual stage T1 cancer on the prostatectomy specimen:

Of the specimens, 38 (86.4%) showed cancer that was in contact with the border of the TURP defect and was likely to represent the cancer sampled by resection.

4. Unsuspected cancers in the specimen:
In addition to the stage T1 cancers, **83 unsuspected tumors were found in 88% of** stage T1a and in **93%** of stage T1b), the majority being non transition zone cancers, **23% being 0.2 cc or more** in volume.

5. Surgical margins:

There were 6 stage T1a and 9 stage T1b cancer with positive surgical margins. Two patients had positive nodes on permanent sections (stage T1b).

6. Post TURP serum PSA:

Post TURP serum PSA levels elevated with increasing residual tumor volumes. PSA of 2.5 ng/ml in 19 of 20 specimens was associated with tumor volumes greater than 0.9 cc. PSA between 1 and 2.5 ng/ml and total volume from 0.0 to 1.88 cc were recorded in 11 cases.

3. CONCLUSIONS.

The findings in this study indicate that the clinical substages T1a and T1b distinguished between small volume versus larger tumors. However, this clinical substaging misclassified 23% of the patients relative to an optimum cutoff value of 1 cc for total volume and 32% relative to a value of 0.6 cc residual cancer.

We conclude that **transurethral sampling of carcinoma** (hence the T1a/T1b substaging system that relies on such material) **cannot predict tumor volume**, either total or residual, **reliably enough for the individual patient.**

Whole cancer grade, like cancer volume, cannot reliably be estimated from transurethral resection tissue samples

This is a very **serious drawback for this subclassification (and the potential management decision based upon it)** since strong evidence has been previously presented that **cancer volume, as well as quantitated histologic grade, is a powerful predictor of prognosis in the individual patient.**

Total cancer volume appears to be the biologi-cal standard for estimating prognosis and is more closely related conceptually to several important aspects of cancer behavior than is residual cancer: an 8 cc carcinoma with a 1 cc residual tumor is is more likely to be biologically aggressive than a 2 cc tumor with the same 1 cc residual cancer.

Findings from other studies suggest that **a tumor of a total volume of 0.2 cc in younger patients and 1 cc in older ones is biologically significant and justifies a radical form of treatment in patients with adequate general health and life expectancy.** By this criterion, t**he majority of stage T1 cancers in this series were of clinical significance, including 6 of 22 stage T1a patients** (27%) with a volume of 1 cc or more.

All of the predictive variables discussed above, total cancer volume, presence of residual cancer, whole cancer grade and presence of undiagnosed additional cancers, **cannot be determined from analysis of the TURP sample.**

Post TURP serum PSA values, and TRUS supplemented with multiple biopsies may in the future hold promises for the accurate staging of incidental carcinoma of the prostate.

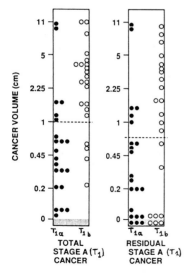

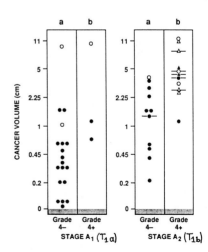

FIG. 1. Relationship between clinical stage (A1 versus A2) and volume of cancer. Volumes are tabulated separately for total cancer (transurethral resection plus residual) and for residual cancer found at prostatectomy. ●, volume of stage A1 cancer (left column). ○, volume of stage A2 cancer (right column). Horizontal line across each tabulation indicates volume that provides best separation between stages A1 and A2 (1.0 cc for total cancer and 0.6 cc for residual cancer).

FIG. 2. Comparison between stages A1 and A2 cancer for volume, grade, extraprostatic tumor (capsule penetration, seminal vesicle invasion or lymph node metastasis) and peripheral zone site of origin. All calculations are for total stage A cancer (transurethral resection plus residual). ● or ▲, no extraprostatic extension. ○ or △, extraprostatic tumor. Grade 4 (or 5) found in total cancer is indicated in right column. △ or ▲, grade 4 was also seen in transurethral resection chips (6 cases, for which 3 were upstaged because of grade 4 in chips). – –, cancer of peripheral zone origin.

Radical prostatectomy for stage T1(A) adenocarcinoma of the prostate: staging errors and their implications for the treatment recommendations and disease outcome.

Horst Zincke, Michael L. Blute, Mark J. Fallen and George Farrow.

J. Urol. 146, 1053,1991.

Basic recommendations regarding stage T1 Prostate Cancer rely on the distinction between stage T1a (A1) (which many authors think should be left untreated) and T1b (A2) (which seems to mandate an active form of treatment). This distinction is mostly based, apart from grade, on the *amount of cancer retrieved at TURP, which is only an indirect estimation of the actual total amount of cancer harbored by the gland (which is likely to be the significant parameter).*

We have studied the pathological specimens from radical prostatectomies for stage T1 tumours in order to assess the correlation between clinical and pathological staging, and to appreciate the implicatons of possible discrepancies.

I. MATERIAL AND METHODS

From 1966 until 1988, 148 patients with unequivocal stage T1 prostate adenocarcinoma underwent bilateral pelvic lymph node dissection and radical prostatectomy. Patients age ranged from 38 to 74 years (mean 63.6 years).

Patients were followed for 1 to 21.5 years (mean 4.6).

Stage T1a was defined as 1 cc of tumour or less or low grade (Mayo 2 or less), and stage T1b as more than 1 cc or high grade (Mayo 3 or more).

Disease progression was identified by biopsy proven local recurrence, abnormal bone scan or an elevated PSA.

Adjuvant hormonal treatment was used in 21 (14%) patients with stage pT1b disease.

Radiation therapy and orchiectomy was used in some other patients with pT3 disease.

II. RESULTS

1. Staging

25% of stage T1a and 9% of T1b had no residual cancer on the specimen.

12% of stage T1a and 29% of stage T1b had stage pT3 on the specimen.

13% of the specimens were margin positive.

2. Clinical grade and pathological stage

None of the 32 patients with clinical grade 1, but 60% of the 20 patients with clinical T1b had pT3 disease.

3. Repeat TURP

It was done in only 14 Patients, 7 T1a and 7 T1b, all of whom had tumour at repeat TURP. Of the 7 patients with clinical stage T1a, 3 were stage pT0, whereas all stage T1b had residual cancer on the radical prostatectomy specimen.

In no instance did repeat TURP help to assess or predict the final pathological stage which varied from pT0 to pT3.

4. Progression

Progression could not be predicted on the clinical stage (T1a vs. T1b) or the pathological stage, at least for the duration of the follow up, except for a highly significant difference between T1a and T1b, if one included an elevated PSA as a criterion for recurrence.

5. Survival

Overall survival in the 148 patients was 92.5%, 73.2% and 59.7% respectively at 5, 10 and 15 years, which is comparable to the expected survival of an age matched control group. Overall survival, and even more so cause-specific survival, was significantly better in stage T1a than in stage T1b patients (Figure 1).

No patients with stage pT0 or pT3c died of cancer (but this may in part be due to the adjuvant treatment that they received in a higher proportion), but 4 of the 62 pT1b did.

5. DNA ploidy

Of the 33 patients who had DNA ploidy measurements, 76% had diploid tumours, and 24% nondiploid tumours.

6. Adjuvant treatment

Of 12 patients with pT3 disease and adjuvant treatment (radiation therapy in 6, hormonotherapy in 6), only one had progression.

V. CONCLUSION

The appropriate treament for stage T1 disease is controversial. The decision to treat agressively depends for most surgeons on the estimation of the local extent or differentiation of the tumour, namely, separation into the classical stage T1a and stage T1b.

The concept that stage T1a disease is innocuous cannot be supported when follow up is extended for a prolonged period. For instance, short term follow up of a group of patients with stage T1a reported disease progression in 2% or less in a classic study by Cantrell : however, when patients with the same disease were followed for a minimum of 8 years, disease progression was observed in 16%. Furthermore *6 of these 8 patients who had progression died within a mean of 2 years.*

This is confirmed by a study at our institution where 4 of 15 young (less than 60 years) patients (26%) with stage T1a tumours followed for 10 to 25 years had disease progression after 9 to 14 years.

These observations suggest that *patients less than 60 years, who have a life expectancy extending beyond 8 to 10 years are at significant risk for progression* and thus are candidates for definitive surgical treatment.

At the present time, clinical separation of stage T1a and stage T1b proves a most difficult undertaking, as demonstrated by the present study. As long as it is so, *it may be prudent not to rely entirely on the traditional criteria of definition of stages T1a and T1b as true predictors of the biological behaviour of the tumour, and offer an active form of treatment to stage T1a patients with a sigificant life expectancy.*

The advent of serum PSA, improvements in TRUS and routine application of DNA ploidy studies may help in the future better identify those tumours that are likely to remain indolent and those which will cause significant morbidity.

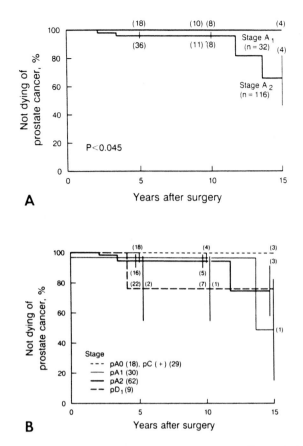

Figure 1. Kaplan-Meier projection of cause-specific survival in 148 patients with clinical stage A (T1) adenocarcinoma of prostate who had bilateral pelvic lymphadenectomy and radical retropubic prostatectomy.

A, according to clinical substage (A1[T1a] versus A2 [T1b]) .

B, according to pathological stage. Numbers in parentheses are numbers of patients still under observation at this interval.

Radiotherapy for Incidental Adenocarcinoma of the Prostate

I.D. Kaplan, M.A. Bagshaw, C.A. Cox, R.S. Cox

Department of Radiation Oncology, Stanford University School of Medicine, Stanford, California, USA

Stage T_1 or *Stage A* (incidental) prostate carcinoma patients are a *heterogeneous group : some never experience disease progression and others have a high incidence of lymph node involvement and die of metastasis* irrespective of treatment.

The *incidence of progression* has been somewhat underestimated in the published series of the literature, but Epstein has found that 16% of patients and Lowe 26% of patients progresed if left untreated. Considering the studies by McNeal et al. demonstrating an interrelationship between tumor bulk, histologic differentiation and metastatic potential, it is *prudent to consider that, given enough time, incidental prostate carcinoma may not be insignificant and can potentially progress to local and/or metastatic disease.*

This series of *85 patients with incidental carcinoma of the prostate* treated with external beam radiation therapy at Stanford University between 1967 and 1988 (22 with focal disease (T1a) and 63 with diffuse disease (T1b)) is the largest such series published: the results of this study can be compared to the results of series using other treatment modalities, therefore contributing to discussions on the preferred management of incidental carcinoma of the prostate, and is helpful as well in an attempt to identify the features of patients with a higher risk of progression that might benefit from an early radical treatment.

RESULTS

The survival of the 22 patients with stage T1a disease did not differ significantly from that of the 63 patients with stage T1b, nor did the survival of either stage differ from the expected survival of a cohort of age-matched individuals (Figure 1). There was no significant difference between stages

Table 1. Carcinoma of the prostate stage T1: current status of patients

	T1a (A1)		T1b (A2)	
	(n)	(%)	(n)	(%)
Alive without tumour	13	59	32	51
Alive with tumour	0	0	6	10
Intercurrent Death	7	32	19	30
Without tumour	6	27	17	27
After prior relapse	1	5	1	2
With local tumour	0	0	1	2
Dead with metastases	2	9	6	10
Total	22	26	63	74

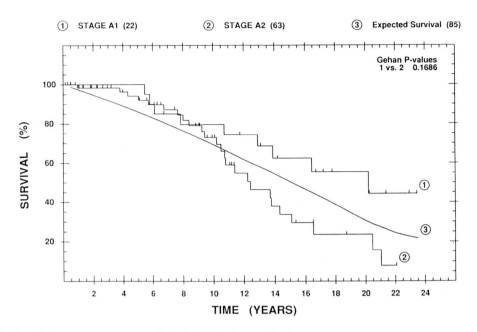

Figure 1. Survival by stage A1 (T1a), A2 (T1b) in prostatic cancer

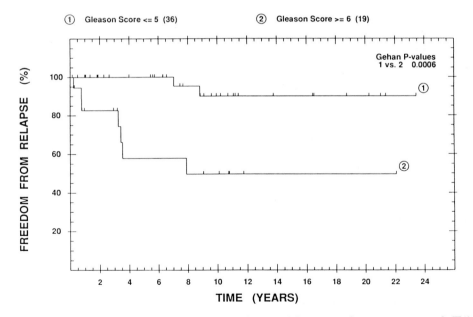

Figure 2. Freedom from relapse by Gleason score (≤ 5, ≥ 6) in prostatic cancer stage A (T1)

T1a and T1b in disease-specific survival or in freedom from relapse. To date, as shown in Table 1, 3 of the 22 patients with stage T1a have relapsed, 2 with metastatic disease. Fourteen of the 63 patients with stage T1b have relapsed. Six are alive with disease at last follow-up; six died of metastases and 1 died of unrelated causes with uncontrolled local disease.

Full pelvic irradiation as opposed to irradiation of the prostatic region only did not significantly improve either survival or freedom from relapse, although the follow-up time is relatively short for those irradiated to the full pelvis.

As far as **parameters predictive of response** to treatment are concerned, we found that older patients tended to relapse more frequently, although the difference with younger patients' relapse rate was not significant. **Gleason grading** was performed in 55 of the 83 patients: it did not correlate with crude or disease specific survival. Gleason score did however correlate with the **relapse rate** (Figure 2)

In conclusion: we have confirmed in this study the negative implication of a high Gleason score (which should be included as a stratification criterion in all future trials) on the relapse rate; we have demonstrated, contrary to a somewhat generally held opinion, **that the relapse rate in the older patients tend to be higher than in the younger ones**, implying that *the former should not be excluded from consideration for treatment on the sole basis of their age.* Our data can give some indication on the effects to be expected from radiotherapy for incidental carcinoma of the prostate, but we are fully aware that the **role of treatment, be it radiotherapy, surgery or other**, for incidental cacinoma of the prostate **can be analyzed only with prospective randomized trials.**

DOCUMENTATION

BAGSHAW MA. Current conflicts in the management of prostatic cancer. Int J Radiat Oncol Biol Phys 12:1721-1727, 1986.

BEYNON LL, BUSUTTIL A, NEWSAM JE, CHISHOLM GD. Incidental carcinoma of the prostate: selection for deferred treatment. Br J Urol 55:733-736, 1983.

EPSTEIN JI, PAULL G, EGGLESTON JC, WALSH PC. Prognosis of untreated stage A1 prostatic carcinoma: a study of 94 cases with extended follow-up. J Urol 136:837-839, 1986.

JOHANSSON JE, ANDERSSON SO, KRUSEMO UB, ADAMI HO, BERGSTROM, R, KRAAZ W. Natural history of localized prostatic cancer: a population-based study in 223 untreated patients. Lancet 8642:799-803, 1989.

LOWE BA, LISTROM MB. Incidental carcinoma of the prostate: an analysis of the predictors of progression. J Urol 140:1340-1344, 1988.

LOWE BA, LISTROM MB. Management of stage A prostate cancer with a high probability of progression. J Urol 140:1345-1347, 1988.

MADSEN PO, GRAVERSEN PH, GASSER TL, CORLE DK. Treatment of localized cancer. Radical prostatectomy versus placebo. A 15 year follow-up. Scand J Urol Nephrol (Suppl) 110:95-100, 1988.

MCNEAL JE. Origin and development of carcinoma in the prostate. Cancer 23:24-34, 1969.

PISTENMA DA, BAGSHAW MA, FREIHA FS. Extended field radiation therapy for prostatic adenocarcinoma. Status report of a limited prospective trial. In: Johnson PE, Samuels ML (eds) Cancer of the genitourinary tract. Raven, New York, pp 229-248, 1979.

II

Stage T2 (B)

Selection of Patients with Stage B (T2) Prostate Cancer for Radical Prostatectomy

Richard G. Middleton,

Division of Urology, University of Utah Center for the Health Sciences, Salt Lake City, Utah, USA

I. DIGITAL RECTAL EXAMINATION: VALUE AND SHORTCOMINGS

A review of Jewett's results illustrates both the value and the shortcomings of digital rectal examination in the staging or selection of patients for what is hoped to be a curative procedure. 27% of Jewett's patients were alive and well without recurrence 15 years after radical prostatectomy. There were 86 of the 103 patients (83%) whose radical prostatectomy specimens showed tumor localized to the prostate. In 17 cases, there was microscopic extension of the tumor to the seminal vesicles, and *no* patient with *seminal vesicle involvement survived 15 years without recurrence of tumor.* Overall, about one third of Jewett's patients with T2a nodules died of cancer, whereas another third died of causes unrelated to prostatic cancer.

Walsh and Jewett reviewed 57 further patients with clinical stage T2a prostate cancer who had radical perineal prostatectomy from 1951 to 1963. Fifteen years later, 51% were alive and well, 17% had died of tumor recurrence, and 32% had died without clinical evidence of recurrent prostatic cancer. The survival of these selected patients with small clinical stage T2 lesions was similar to that of similar-age white men in the general population. Similar survival rates after radical prostatectomy for small (and usually low-grade) T2 tumor nodules were reported by other authors.

Stage T2a (B1)

These experiences point up that in dealing with the clinical T2a prostatic nodule understaging is common, probably both because the examiner sometimes fails to appreciate the full extent of the palpable tumor induration and because the examiner cannot hope to feel microscopic tumor extension to the seminal vesicles and beyond, the recognition of tumor extension into the seminal vesicles being of great importance for the prognosis.

Stage T2b-c (B2-3)

For clinical T2b (stage B2), or T2c (B3) involving more than half of the prostate, the problem of defining the extent of the tumor accurately by rectal examination is compounded. Even the experienced urologist may have a difficult time distinguishing the clinical T2b-c lesion from the stage T3 (C) tumor that extends outside the prostate capsule. Jewett, in his radical perineal prostatectomy series up to 1951, reported that approximately 50% of those patients with T2b-c (large B) lesions clinically had seminal vesicle invasion on microscopic examination, and only 18 per cent survived without recurrence for 15 years. Interestingly, though, of those patients with T2b lesions and negative seminal vesicles, 30% lived 15 years or more.

On the basis of many reports, it seems clear

that digital rectal examination for staging is even less reliable with large T2b lesions than it is with T2a (B1), or small, nodules. In some series, as many as 40% to 60% of patients judged to have T2b tumors actually have pathologic stage pT3 or N+ tumors. *Selection of patients to undergo radical prostatectomy with curative intent requires more accurate staging measures.*

II. PELVIC LYMPH NODE ASSESSMENT

Currently available imaging techniques have not proved reliable in demonstrating the presence of pelvic nodal metastasis in clinical stage T2 prostatic cancer. Lymphangiography, CT scanning, MRI, and ultrasonography have been unsatisfactory for lymph node evaluation when a radical prostatectomy is under consideration.

The need for surgical staging by lymph node dissection and frozen-section histologic examination is mandatory.

Bilateral pelvic lymphadenectomy is carried out for staging at the beginning of the operative procedure. The surgeon should remove nodes for examination beginning on the same side as the prostate nodule. Nodes if *enlarged or hard*, are examined by frozen section. If lymph nodes are *unremarkable grossly*, representative nodes are examined histologically by frozen section.

When lymph nodes are found to be *free* of tumor, radical prostatectomy is carried out. When *nodal metastasis* is discovered, *radical prostatectomy with curative intent seems unreasonable*. However, one can justify proceeding with the radical prostatectomy if the operation is considered to be part of a *clinical protocol* using combinations of therapeutic measures for the purpose of tumor control or suppression.

The *incidence* of tumor extension to lymph nodes in clinical stage T2 prostate carcinoma depends on tumor size and grade.

Table 1. Number (%) of pelvic node metastasis by Gleason grade and clinical stage

STAGE	LOW GRADE (GLEASON 2–4)	MODERATE GRADE (GLEASON 5–7)	HIGH GRADE (GLEASON 8–10)	TOTAL
B1 (T2a)	2/53 (4)	13/94 (14)	3/9 (33)	18/156 (12)
B2 (T2b)	5/27 (18)	29/106 (27)	9/21 (43)	43/154 (28)
Total	7/80 (9)	42/200 (21)	12/20 (60)	61/310 (20)

Table 2. Survival after radical prostatectomy in paitents with negative pelvic nodes

CLINICAL STAGE	ALIVE (%)	ALIVE WITH NO EVIDENCE OF RECURRENCE (%)	DIED OF PROSTATE CANCER (%)
5 Years			
B1 (T2a)	43/44 (98)	40/44 (91)	0 (0)
B2 (T2b)	52/58 (90)	47/58 (81)	4 (7)
Total	95/102 (93)	87/102 (85)	4 (4)
10 Years			
B1 (T2a)	30/38 (79)	20/38 (53)	5/38 (13)
B2 (T2b)	18/30 (60)	15/30 (50)	7/30 (23)
Total	48/68 (71)	35/68 (51)	12/68 (18)

Our experience with 452 pelvic lymphadenectomies has been reported from the University of Utah (Table I).

Only 2 of 53 patients with low-grade *T2a tumor* nodules had positive pelvic nodes. The incidence of nodal involvement increased to 14% and 33% in moderately differentiated and poorly differentiated clinical T2a tumors, respectively.

With *clinical T2b tumor* nodules the incidence of positive nodes ranged from 18% with well-differentiated primaries to 43% with poorly differentiated lesions.

From the University of Utah, we also have *survival rate data* for those patients with clinically localized or T2 tumors who were proved by staging pelvic lymphadenectomy to have negative lymph nodes before radical prostatectomy (Table 2). Our experience with radical prostatectomy in these selected patients has shown excellent survival rates and a low recurrence rate at 5 and 10 years. Of the 10 patients who had clinical T1b or T2 cancers and microscopic tumor in the seminal vesicles, only 5 were free of recurrence at 5 years.

III. PROSTATE-SPECIFIC ANTIGEN AND ACID PHOSPHATASE

Useful markers for prostate cancer are prostatic acid phosphatase and prostate-specific antigen.

1. Prostatic acid phosphatase

A significant question is *whether an elevated prostatic acid phosphatase level predictably signifies extracapsular extension of the prostate tumor*. Reviewing cases of clinically localized prostate cancer treated with bilateral node dissection and radical retropubic prostatectomy, Salo and Rannikko found that an elevation in either the enzymatic or the radioimmunoassay for determining prostatic acid phosphatase was

an indication of extracapsular tumor spread with a *specificity of 100%*. Thus, *if prostatic acid phosphatase is elevated, there is a very high probability of extracapsular extension.*

In this report, the sensitivity was only 37% and 6 per cent for the radioimmunoassay and enzymatic methods for prostatic acid phosphatase determination, respectively, indicating that a *normal prostatic acid phosphatase does not exclude extracapsular tumor extension.*

The *average* serum prostatic acid phosphatase level for *intracapsular cancer* was 1.4 ± 0.8 units, with a range of 0.4 to 3.0 units.

For *extracapsular disease*, the average prostatic acid phosphatase was 3.5 ± 2.8 units, with a range of 0.8 to 9.9. *The level of 3.0 units was selected as a value above which one could confidently predict extracapsular tumor extension* (normal ranges vary with methods of determination). It can be seen that there is much overlap in the prostatic acid phosphatase values encountered with intracapsular and extracapsular cancer. It is known that with prostatic acid phosphatase elevated to the upper limit of normal and into the low abnormal range, the risk of extracapsular tumor extension increases significantly. With markedly elevated prostatic acid phosphatase, *twice the upper limit of normal and beyond, extracapsular spread is virtually certain.*

2. Prostate-specific antigen

Prostate-specific antigen is another prostatic protein. Because this marker is produced by normal and hyperplastic prostates, prostate-specific antigen has not been found reliable as a screening test for prostate cancer. Values for men with normal prostates are nearly always under 4 ng/ml. After total prostatectomy, the prostate-specific antigen value should drop to below 0.3 ng/ml.

Barak and coworkers noted that in a group of apparently *healthy men*, all had prostate-specific antigen levels of less than 6 ng/ml, and 90 % had levels lower than 2 ng/ml.

In a *urologic population* where patients have associated benign hyperplasia, these investigators suggested that *about 10 ng/ml is the upper limit of normal.*

Their mean value for clinical stage *T2 prostate cancer* was 45 ng/ml; 67 ng/ml was the mean value for *stage T3 (C)* disease, and 292 ng/ml was the mean level for patients with *stage M+ (D$_2$)* prostate cancer. There were significant overlaps.

This work agrees with other studies, which have shown that fewer than 15% of patients with benign hyperplasia have prostate-specific antigen levels greater than 10 ng/ml, and rarely is benign hyperplasia associated with a level greater than 20 ng/ml. Stamey and associates reported that no patient with positive nodes in their experience had a prostate-specific antigen below 10 ng/ml. For those patients whose prostate-specific antigen was greater than 50 ng/ml, two thirds had positive lymph nodes, and 90% had seminal vesicle involvement. There was *no difference in prostate-specific antigen levels between those who had tumor confined to the prostate and those with slight capsular penetration.*

Reports associate small increases in prostate-specific antigen with increasing prostate size, acute prostatitis, and the onset of urinary retention.

Prostate-specific antigen can be a useful guide in the staging of prostate cancer, but it is not an absolute indicator. There is no prostate-specific antigen level that definitely indicates that the tumor is localized to the prostate, nor is there a level that surely indicates tumor extension outside the prostate. Although prostate-specific antigen can be used as a rough indicator of the stage of prostate cancer, it has been more reliable as an indicator of the response to treatment in a patient with known prostate cancer.

IV. TUMOR PLOIDY

There is increasing evidence that the determination of nuclear ploidy of prostate tumor cells can be helpful in the preoperative assessment of patients and in estimating prognosis. Ploidy does not correlate predictably with tumor grade. Tumors that are diploid are associated with a much lower incidence of extracapsular extension than are those with an aneuploid pattern. Also tumor recurrence and the rate of progression are reported to be much greater in aneuploid than in diploid tumors. *Currently, ploidy does not play much of a role in the selection of patients for radical prostatectomy,* but with more experience, we may be more likely to follow nonoperatively the patient with a diploid T2a tumor or recommend prostatectomy in a patient of borderline age whose tumor is aneuploid and therefore likely to progress.

III. TRANSRECTAL ULTRASOUND AS AN ADJUNCT TO DIGITAL RECTAL EXAMINATION

Digital rectal examination has long been the standard for detection, presumptive diagnosis, and clinical staging of prostate cancer. *Ultrasound can be helpful and complementary to digital rectal examination.* Staging of prostate cancer by ultrasound screening is an area of emerging importance. Areas of extracapsular extension can be detected with biopsies obtained precisely from the extracapsular sites. *Guided biopsies of the seminal vesicles* are becoming feasible prior to radical prostatectomy. Careful ultrasound scanning with biopsies of suspect areas beyond the pros-

Table 3. Average number of years of life expectancy in white American men, 1986 (National center for health statistics)

AGE	AVERAGE YEARS REMAINING
65	14.8
70	11.7
75	9.1
80	6.9

tate must be correlated with whole-mount examination of radical prostatectomy specimens to define the value of transrectal ultrasound in the routine staging of clinically localized prostate cancer.

V. LIFE EXPECTANCY AND TUMOR PROGRESSION

In an *elderly man* with other life-threatening diseases, a small low grade prostate tumor may be a trivial matter. Certainly, many tumor nodules progress slowly. But how does one objectively decide when the patient is at risk from the cancer and recommend radical prostatectomy, assuming that the tumor is localized?

Whitmore followed patients with *clinical stage T2 prostate tumors* nonoperatively. His results are interesting. Two thirds of his patients showed no apparent progression with a mean follow-up exceeding 6 years. However, one third had progression of the disease with a mean of 59 months of follow-up.

Hanash and coworkers reported that only 19% of patients with stage T2 (mostly T2b) cancers treated conservatively survived 5 years.

Clearly, a patient with a *T2b lesion* is at real risk without surgery if his expected survival otherwise will exceed 5 years. The patient with a *T2a nodule* (especially if low grade) is not at much risk for a 5-year period, but with a 10-year projected longevity,

even the low grade T2a nodule can be a serious risk to life.

For the American white male in 1986, the average number of years of *life expectancy* is listed by age in Table 3. These data can be useful in judging whether a patient is better served by radical prostatectomy or conservative monitoring.

In the *elderly patient*, the urologist certainly may elect to *follow the tumor* without definitely deciding on operative versus conservative treatment. Regular assessment by rectal examination and prostate-specific antigen determination will help to identify the aggressive lesion. Flow cytometry offers the opportunity to identify the lesion that is likely to be indolent and also to recognize that tumor which probably will have a rapid growth rate. The place of transrectal ultrasound in monitoring the progression of tumor is under investigation.

DOCUMENTATION

ANDRIOLE GL, KAVOUSSI LR, TORRENCE RJ, et al: Transrectal ultrasonography in the diagnosis and staging of carcinoma of the prostate. J. Urol., 140:758, 1988

BARAK M, MECA Y, LURIE A, et al: Evaluation of prostatic specific antigen as a marker for adenocarcinoma of the prostate. J Lab Clin Med 1 13:598 1989

BUAMAH PK, JOHNSON P, SKILLEN AW: Comparative study of the clinical usefulness of prostatic specific antigen and prostatic acid phosphatase in prostatic disease. Br J Urol 62:581, 1988.

DEJTER SW, CUNNINGHAM RE, NOGUCHI PD, et al: Prognostic significance of DNA ploidy in carcinoma of the prostate. Urology 33:361, 198915. Hudson MA, Bahnson RR, Catalona WJ: Clinical use of prostate specific antigen in patients with prostate cancer. J Urol 142:1011, 1989.

JEWETT HJ: The present status of radical prostatectomy for stages A and B prostate cancer. Urol Clin North Am 2: 105, 1975.

MIDDLETON RG SMITH JA JR, MELZER RB, et al:

Patient survival and local recurrence rate following radical prostatectomy for prostatic carcinoma. J Urol 136:422, 1986.

SMITH JA JR, SEAMAN JP, GLEIDMAN JB, et al: Pelvic lymph node metastasis from prostatic cancer: Influence of tumor grade and stage in 452 consecutive patients. J Urol 130:290, 1983.

STAMEY TA, KABALIN JN: Prostate specific antigen in the diagnosis and treatment of adenocarcinoma of the prostate I: Untreated patients. J Urol 141:1070, 198926. Walsh PC, Jewett HJ: Radical surgery for prostate cancer. Cancer 45:1906 1980.

WHITMORE WF Jr: Natural history and staging of prostate cancer. Urol Clin North Am 11:205, 1984.

WINKLER HZ, RAINWATER LM, MYERS RP, et al: Stage D1 prostatic adenocarcinoma: Significance of nuclear DNA ploidy patterns studied by flow cystometry. Mayo Clin Proc 63:103, 1988.

Radiation Therapy for Localized Prostate Cancer: Long-term Follow-up

Malcolm A. Bagshaw, MD, Richard S. Cox, PhD, Ira and Joyce E. Ramback.
Department of Radiation Oncology, Stanford University School of Medicine, Stanford, California

The lack of a randomized controlled study makes it difficult to establish the true efficacy of irradiation and its ability to sterilize prostatic cancer. The long natural history of many prostatic cancers, the inability to assess the clonogenic viability of apparently residual cancer in post-therapeutic biopsy specimens, and the fact that many elderly patients with a diagnosis of prostatic cancer who succumb to either the neoplasm or some intercurrent disease are rarely submitted to postmortem examination make it extremely difficult to document the true outcome after any treatment in this disease.

It is the purpose of this discussion to examine what may be deduced regarding the radiocurability of prostatic cancer from the analysis of long-term follow-up data. The substantial experience collected at Stanford over the past 34 years will be used as a model.

I. MATERIALS AND METHODS

1. Patient Profile

Definitive irradiation of prostatic carcinoma with external-beam radiation started at Stanford in 1956.

Nineteen per cent of the Stanford patients with stage T2a and T2b disease and 56% of those with stage T3 disease had *lymph nodes histopathologically positive for tumor.*

The treatment regimen for nearly all patients included 7000 rad in 7 weeks to the prostate region and 5000 rad in 7 weeks to the first-echelon lymph nodes.

Few patients have been lost to follow-up, and those who have been were censored at the time of last contact at whatever disease status was known.

2. Follow-up Routine

The *follow-up routine* included visits at 1 4, 8, and 12 months after radiotherapy, followed by visits at 6-month intervals to 5 years and one visit per year thereafter. Follow-up visits included an interim history and performance of an abbreviated physical examination focusing on the status of the skeletal system and the lymphatic system and a digital rectal examination.

Blood was drawn for PAP and later PSA measurements.

Bone scans were ordered only if there was a clinical indication.

Biopsies of the primary site were obtained only if advancing disease was suspected as manifested by digital rectal examination, escalating prostate-specific antigen values, or local symptomatology. Occasionally, they were obtained by the referring urologist at his or her discretion.

II. RESULTS

1. Statistical Presentation

Actuarial curves for the various groups were calculated by the Kaplan and Meier method.

Concerning staging information, the M categories have been omitted, because only patients who showed no evidence of distant metastases were included in these data. The N (lymph node) status also is omitted because it was unknown for the majority of patients although in a subgroup of surgically staged patients, 19% with stage T2 and 56% with stage T3 disease had surgically proved adenopathy.

2. Survival

a) Overall survival curves (Figure 1) such as these in which death from all causes is scored tend to dilute the impact of the treatment on survival because cancer of the prostate is a relatively chronic neoplasm and occurs late in life, and there are many competing causes of death. Nevertheless, note that there is a systematic reduction in survival as stage increases; i.e., survival diminishes with time as a function of the clinical stage. This, of course, is characteristic of most forms of cancer and is compatible with the radiobiology of tumor response.

It is difficult to appreciate from studying Figure 1, but 126 patients survived beyond 15 years, and only 15 died of metastatic disease beyond 15 years. Thirty-five died of intercurrent illness beyond 15 years without clinical evidence of prostatic cancer, and 76 patients are still living.

b) Figure 2 depicts the **disease-specific survival** (cause-specific survival). It shows a statistically significant difference between each of the stages. Although there are a few deaths beyond the 15th year, as noted above for overall survival, there are a large number of survivors beyond that milestone.

c) Figure 3 demonstrates **freedom from relapse** (FFR). This measure appears to provide the *most persuasive demonstration of the efficacy of irradiation* in the treatment of prostatic cancer. In this group of patients, relapse of any type is scored as failure, that is, either failure of control at the primary site or the identification of distant metastases.

Also note that the slope of the FFR curves diminishes with time, indicating that in time, a cohort of patients remains that is **no longer relapsing.** This is in contrast to overall survival displayed in Figure 1, in which, although there is some flattening of the survival curves with time, the effect is not nearly as obvious as shown for FFR in Figure 3.

d) Figure 4 shows the *time course of clinical local control* for each primary tumor stage. As expected, local failure increased with advancing stage except for T3b, in which the curve is paradoxical, indicating that because of the severity of the disease, death from metastatic disease preceded local failure. Figure 4 demonstrates the **value of irradiation of the primary tumor even if long-term cure is not achieved.**

e) Figure 5 demonstrates the **survival and disease-specific survival** for all patients with nodular disease treated at Stanford who *might reasonably have been considered candidates for radical prostatectomy*. This group of patients includes all those who had nodular disease confined to one lateral lobe. Note that the maximum follow-up period *extends beyond 22 years* and that the overall survival was 45 per cent at 15 years, only 5 per cent less than the expected survival of an age-matched cohort of Californian men. This is *remarkably close to the expected survival* when one considers that *all histopathologic grades* were included, the *status of the lymph nodes was unknown* for these patients, and on the basis of previous data obtained

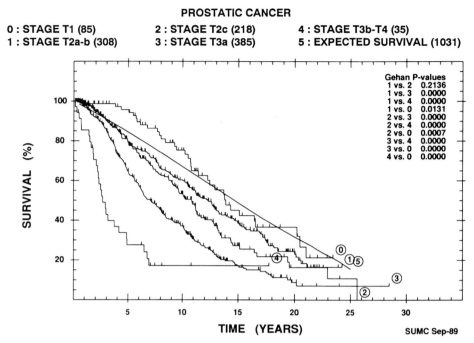

Figure 1. Survival curves as a function of clinical stage. A downward step represents death from any cause; an upward tick represents a patient surviving at last follow-up and censored at the time indicated by the abscissa. Patient may or may not have residual or metastatic cancer. Number in parenthesis is the number of patients in each group.

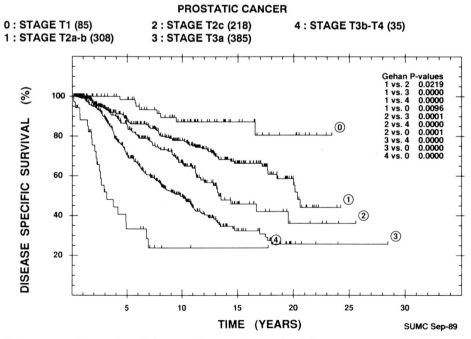

Figure 2. Disease-specific survival. A downward step indicates death from prostate cancer; an upward tick represents a patient who either died of intercurrent disease without evidence of prostatic cancer or was alive at the time of last follow-up; patient may or may not have had cancer at that time.

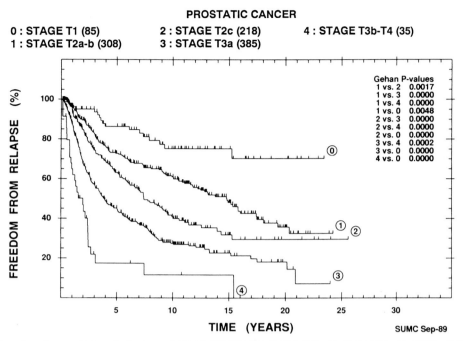

Figure 3. Freedom from relapse. A downward step indicates the first evidence of recurrence, either at the primary site or a metastatic site, as detected by clinical observation or a positive biopsy. An upward tick represents a patient who was either observed disease free or died after being disease free at the time of last observation.

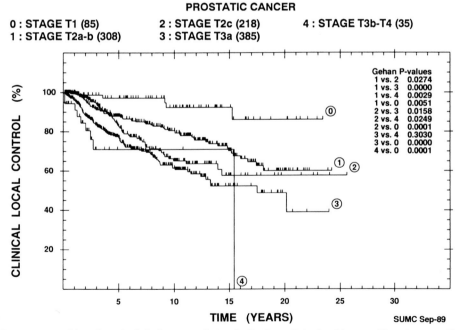

Figure 4. Time course of local control. A downward step indicates clinical evidence of local regrowth after initial regression of tumor or after an initial showing of no evidence of local neoplasm. An upward tick represents a patient who either demonstrated no clinical evidence of local tumor at last follow-up or died without clinical evidence of local neoplasm. Patient could have had evidence of metastatic tumor either while living or at death. Local control is paradoxically high for stage T_4 because many patients die of metastatic disease before lack of local control is manifest.

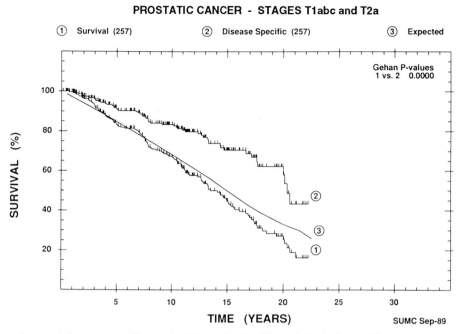

Figure 5. Survival and disease-specific survival for patients with nodular lesions, either apparently confined to one lobe (T₁a, T₁b, T₁c) or confined to one lobe with distortion of the capsule (T₂a), and unknown node status.

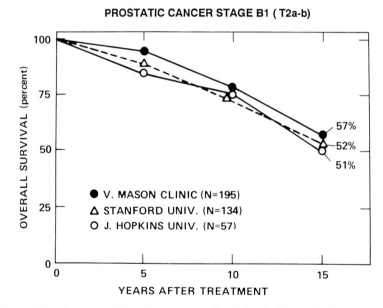

Figure 6. Comparison of long-term survival rates among patients treated by radical surgery or definitive irradation. Long-term survival of patients in stage T2a-b (B1) treated by radiation therapy in the Stanford University series (134 patients; open triangles) and those treated by radical prostatectomy in the series at the Johns Hopkins Hospital (57 patients open circles) and the Virginia Mason Medical Center (195 patients; solid circles) is presented. (Wiliam U. Shipley, MD, personal communication, 1986.)

146

by surgical staging, at least 14 per cent of the patients in these staging categories had metastatic spread to regional lymph nodes. Figure 6 also demonstrates that the disease-specific survival at 15 years was 70 per cent.

f) Figure 6 compares *three well-known series of patients with apparently localized carcinoma*, each followed beyond 15 years: two treated by *radical surgery*, and one by *definitive radiation*. In assessing these data, one must recognize that they were collected over a long period of time at three different institutions (Johns Hopkins University, Stanford University, and the Virginia Mason Clinic) using three different staging systems. It is impossible to know whether the three series are comparable. It is clear from inspection of Figure 10 that there was *no difference in outcome that could be attributed to the treatment modality.* Moreover, it appeared that the expectation of survival for 15 years was approximately 50 per cent irrespective of the treatment modality, or equivalent to that of an age-matched cohort of Californian men (solid line, Figure 1).

III. DISCUSSION

1) It has been shown here that *long-term survival rates* indistinguishable from those expected from an age-matched peer group may be anticipated after x-irradiation in appropriately selected patients with prostatic cancer.

2) Selection factors that have been demonstrated to impact on longevity include *clinical stage, histopathologic grade*—especially as characterized by the Gleason system—and the *status of the lymph nodes.*

3) The optimum treatment for such patients depends on proper case selection, with *prudent consideration of factors other*

than survival alone, because survival compatible with that expected for an age-matched peer group appears likely in either case.

Cofactors relevant to selection of the appropriate treatment modality include age, general health status, relative morbidity, and patient preference.

4) *The issue of choosing between surgery or irradiation* in well-selected cases is not as great in our opinion as is the issue of choosing patients for surgery whose disease is truly resectable.

In the past, preoperative understaging has been common and frequently associated with incomplete resection.

Precise staging is not as critical before radiation therapy because generous treatment margins sufficient to include capsular penetration, periprostatic involvement, seminal vesicle invasion or, in some cases, lymph nodes, are standard.

5) To be sure, long-term survival after irradiation diminishes systematically with more advanced disease, but it *does not fall to zero even in the most advanced stage.*

IV. SUMMARY

1) For patients with clinical stage *T2a-b* disease (nodular disease that did not exceed involvement of one lateral lobe), *survival was only 5% less at 15 years than for the age-matched group of Californian men.* This was in spite of the fact that the lymph node status and the true incidence of capsular penetration were unknown. Moreover, the patients were not stratified by histopathologic grade or by either acid phosphatase or prostate-specific antigen values. If one were to restrict the patients to those with intermediate and low Gleason scores, normal acid phosphatase, and low prostate-specific antigen values, it is likely that there

would have been no difference between the survival of those with prostatic cancer and their age-matched peers.

2) As one deviates from these conservative selection criteria and includes *patients with more advanced stages, the likelihood of achieving 15-year survival diminishes*.

3) With radiation treatment, however, patients whose disease, by clinical examination, *extends beyond the prostate and who seem too advanced for radical prostatectomy* still may have a *20% to 30% chance of 15-year survival.*

DOCUMENTATION

ALLAIN YM, BOLLA M, DOUCHEZ J, et al: Cancer de la prostate: Résultats de la radiothérapie: Étude inter-centres. Bull Cancer Paris 72:559, 1985.

BAGSHAW MA: Current conflicts in the management of prostatic cancer. Int J Radiat Oncol Biol Physics12:1721,1986.

BAGSHAW MA: External beam irradiation of prostatic cancer. In Coffey DS, Resnick Ml, Dorr FA, et al (eds): A Multidisciplinary Analysis of Controversies in the Management of Prostate Cancer. New York, Plenum Publishing, p. 85, 1988.

BAGSHAW MA, COX RS, RAY GR: Status of radiation treatment of prostate cancer at Stanford University. NCI Monographs 7:47, 1988.

BAGSHAW MA, KAPLAN HS, SAGERMAN RH: Linear accelerator supervoltage radiotherapy VII: Carcinoma of the prostate. Radiology 85:121, 1965.

The Case for No Initial Treatment of Localized Prostate Cancer

Philip H. Smith, FRCS*

Department of Urology, St. James's University Hospital, Leeds, United Kingdom

At first sight, it seems illogical to consider deferred treatment in any condition whether malignant or not. Further thought, however, suggests that, particularly in the elderly, **conditions may be monitored rather than treated** if the risk of treatment is high, the toxicity considerable, or the likely benefit small. For example a diagnosis of "superficial" bladder cancer that invades the lamina propria (category T1 disease) merits local treatment to control symptoms but is not usually an indication for early cystectomy despite the recognition that a significant percentage of these patients will, if they live long enough, ultimately develop invasive bladder cancer.

If localized prostatic cancer is considered in the same way, it becomes necessary to be aware of its unusual **natural history** and to understand the **limitations** and the **hazards** of any treatment proposed before assuming that immediate treatment is mandatory: i.e., that it will undoubtedly be of benefit to the individual patient—or even, on balance, of benefit to patients as a group.

I. NATURAL HISTORY

The key to this issue is the incidence of latent cancer, which rises from 5% to 10% at the age of 50 years to 20% to 30% in those over 70 years of age. Dr. Madsen observed that there are 55 million men over the age of 50 years in the USA, implying that at least **5 million will have prostatic cancer**, the vast majority of cases being undiagnosed, as **only 100,000** new cases are **reported each year**. Of these, **26,000 die of prostatic cancer**. Clearly, **the vast majority** of people with prostatic cancer **never develop symptoms from their disease.**

Of patients with concidentally diagnosed prostate cancer, 8% develop metastases within 10 years and that 2% die from the disease, whereas in those with solitary palpable nodules within the prostate, 30% develop metastases within 5 years and 20% die from the disease. In those with positive regional lymph nodes, 50% develop distant metastases after 2 years and 80% after 5 years, and half the patients are dead within 5 years (Studer).

Once a suspect lesion is found, checked by ultrasound, and confirmed by needle biopsy, both surgeon and patient have a dilemma. The simplest, and from the clinician's view, the safest clinical and medicolegal approach is to advise **radical therapy** (whether this is by radical prostatectomy or by radiotherapy).

The **essential question** to be considered here is **whether such therapy is justified or indeed justifiable**.

Let us assume that the 55 million men over the age of 50 years have an average life expectancy of 20 years. Ten per cent have prostatic cancer, but the condition will be diagnosed in only 100,000 of these patients each year—2 million in all over the average life span. Of this 2 million, 26% (520,000) will die of the cancer. Assuming that all cases could be diagnosed, any therapy offered would be **overtreatment for almost 90% of the patients.**

Once this point is grasped, it becomes possible to take a new look at the overall picture of prostatic cancer, whose course is far different from that of many of the other common solid tumors.

The task of the surgeon is to understand the significance of latent cancer, to recognize the importance of histologic grade, and to take account of the fact that the progression of disease in many patients, even in those in whom the primary lesion is clinically apparent, is frequently measured in terms of years rather than months of symptom-free survival.

Most surgeons accept that a **uniform therapeutic strategy will not suit all cases** but remain uncertain about which criteria should be dominant in guiding them in their choice of treatment. In this tumor, the search is for a subset of patients who both need and will benefit from treatment.

II. LIMITATIONS OF PROPOSED TREATMENTS

1. Sucess rate of radical treatment

a) Cases with a good prognosis

All urologists recognize that the **extent** of **spread** of disease at diagnosis and the **grade** of the tumor are vital in determining the prognosis. It is this recognition that has resulted in attempts to make the diagnosis while the tumor is small and the patient asymptomatic.

It is, therefore, natural for the surgeon to seek to treat the patient whose tumor is **well differentiated** at a stage **when it is also small.**

Unfortunately for this view, it is in this group of patients that tumor progression may occur slowly if at all. Gleason has analyzed the combined prognostic significance of grade and stage and concluded that a patient with a well-differentiated nodule in the prostate that is less than 1.5 cm in diameter and Gleason grade 4 to 8, has very little chance of dying of his tumor, whether treated or not. This is the first challenge facing both the surgeon and the radiotherapist, because **they must demonstrate in this group of patients that active treatment with its complications is superior to surveillance with treatment on progression.** So far, no trials have yet demonstrated that intervention is preferable to surveillance.

a) Cases with a poor prognosis

The real task facing both the surgeon and the radiotherapist, however, is to demonstrate their capacity to control the disease in the patient in whom the **tumor is likely to progress;** i.e., the patient with a poorly differentiated lesion. All the evidence so far suggests that radical prostatectomy is unlikely to be of assistance to this group of patients. Elder and associates noted that **radical prostatectomy had little to offer the patient with a poorly differentiated T2b lesion, and Jewett believed that no patient with a G3 cancer** should be treated by radical prostatectomy. It is probable that **radiotherapy is of equally little help** to this group of patients, but it is less easy to be certain, as such patients are usually treated without prior lymph node resection. Because the nodes are positive in patients with poorly differentiated tumors in 40% or more of cases, the surgeon would have rejected these cases even before undertaking his operation. Inevitably, therefore, the series are not comparable.

The statistics show a marked increase in the involvement of the pelvic lymph nodes as the tumor increases in stage and as it becomes less differentiated. It is also recognized that there is little point in proceeding with radical prostatectomy in patients whose lymph nodes are positive, because the development of metastatic disease outside the pelvis is likely to follow within a few years.

It may be argued that the general use of preprostatectomy lymph node dissection would allow that subset of patients with **poorly differentiated tumors but negative lymph nodes to benefit from therapy by excision of their apparently localized disease.** Unfortunately, however, patients with localized disease that is poorly differentiated have a high incidence of capsular involvement not expected at the time of surgery suggesting that the true benefit will be minimal. Moreover, such benefit will be gained at considerable financial outlay, which will have been in vain for many patients who either did not need the operation or who could not benefit from it.

2. Financial Cost

The cost of providing treatment varies from center to center and from year to year. However, figures taken from the State of California in 1984 show that both radical surgery and radiotherapy are expensive with an average of $14,000 for radical surgery and $6,000 for radiotherapy.

3. Toxicity

Neither surgeon nor radiotherapist likes to consider that his preferred therapy may be harmful to the patient.

A great step forward in this connection has been the development of the **nerve-sparing radical prostatectomy** by Dr. Walsh, allowing sexual function to be retained in more than half the patients subjected to radical prostatectomy. Despite this improvement, however, the operation is not without its morbidity.

External beam radiotherapy is less immediately traumatic than surgical intervention but does have the disadvantage of damaging the rectal mucosa and the base of the bladder. Patients inevitably experience temporary frequency and urgency of micturition and some bowel dysfunction: as many as 10% also have long-term complications, including proctitis and ischemic fibrosis of the rectum, hematuria, contracted bladder and urethral stricture.

III. MAKING THE DECISION

These observations seem to me to argue strongly against population screening and **against radical surgery or radical radiotherapy in the absence of symptoms or at least of evidence of progression.** These considerations therefore argue in favor of surveillance after diagnosis until such time as evidence of progression is seen whether by rectal examination, transrectal ultrasound, changes in biochemical markers, or the development of symptoms. At that stage, the patient clearly has a lesion that is progressive and is then in a good position to decide which form of therapy he wishes to have. Dr Whitmore observed: considering the frequency with which watchful waiting has been used in the management of stage T2 cancer, usually with endocrine therapy on progression, there is a dearth of information. Limited evidence suggests that the overall 15 year survival rates are similar to those of radical excision or irradiation. He also noted that in his view, and from his long experience, there was little evidence that **cure is possible for those in whom it is necessary or that cure is necessary in those for whom it is possible.**

SUMMARY

This contribution summarizes the evidence from the natural history and pathology of this disease that, given the high incidence of latent cancer, a policy of **radical treatment at diagnosis will represent overtreatment in the majority of cases**. As yet neither radical prostatectomy nor radical radiotherapy has been shown to be **effective in managing the poorly differentiated tumor** in the patient with "localized" disease. For the patient with well-differentiated disease there is little evidence that early treatment is mandatory, because the majority of these patients will not die of prostatic cancer.

The adoption of a policy of **diagnosis followed by active surveillance** would spare many patients the hazard and discomfort of a major operation or of a course of radiotherapy, would minimize expenditure, and would ensure that treatment was given only to those patients in whom progression had been demonstrated. Such an approach is almost certain to be as effective as treatment at diagnosis. Confirmation of this view is likely to be obtained from the existing studies of immediate versus delayed orchiectomy or LHRH therapy currently being undertaken by the Urological Working Party of the Medical Research Council in the United Kingdom and the Urological Group of the EORTC within Europe.

DOCUMENTATION

GOODMAN CM, BUSUTTIL A, CHISHOLM GD: Age, size and grade of tumour predict prognosis in incidentally diagnosed carcinoma of the prostate. Br J Urol 62:576-580, 1988

JEWETT HJ: Radical perineal prostatectomy for palpable, clinically localized, nonobstructive cancer: Experience at the Johns Hopkins Hospital 1909-1963. J Urol 124:492-494, 1980

WHITMORE WF Jr: Overview: Historical and contemporary. NCI Monogr 7:7-11, 1988

The Patient, Disease Status, and Treatment Options for Localized Prostate Cancer: Stages T2a (B1) and T2b (B2)

M. Bazinet, H. W. Herr

Department of Urology, The Sloan Kettering Memorial Cancer Institute, New York, USA

I. INTRODUCTION

There is no disputing that the optimal management of patients with stage T2 prostatic carcinoma is the most uncertain if not the most controversial issue in modern urologic oncology. The present uncertainty can be related to three major factors:

a) the *variable* and *unpredictable natural survival* of the host determined by competing causes of death in a patient population that is generally older than 50 years of age;

b) the *unpredictable natural course of localized disease* as reflected by the independent variables of growth rate, metastatic potential, and therapeutic responsiveness, effectiveness of surgery and irradiation, or combinations thereof, in producing favorable results in some patients;

c) the *relative effectiveness of different methods of treatment* has been and remains clouded by a constantly changing array of clinical staging techniques, selection criteria for treatment, and definitions of response, and by the general absence of satisfactory control data.

Despite the real and well-founded uncertainties regarding "the best form of treatment," it has not prevented the development of strong individual or institutional prejudices, and these, rather than convincing evidence of therapeutic superiority, have helped determine patterns of treatment.

II. NATURAL HISTORY OF STAGE T2 PROSTATIC CANCER

There are at least two features of prostatic cancers that influence its natural history: growth rate and metastatic potential.

1. Growth Rate

The growth rates of histologically similar prostatic carcinomas show considerable variation in their clinical behavior. The MSKCC experience in a select small number of patients with stage T2 disease indicates that the growth of some prostatic lesions is very slow. On the other hand, not all prostatic nodules behave so benignly. Such tumors in some patients have progressed rapidly both locally and systemically despite treatment. For practical purposes, the clinician has no simple and reliable way of estimating growth rate in evaluating a patient's disease at a single point in time. Serial observations of changes in tumor size with time give some indication of growth rate, but this is obviously not uniformly practical in the clinical situation. Although tumor grade may be the best method currently available to estimate the growth rate of a given tumor, clearly better methods are needed to assess the functional capacity of prostatic tumor cells to grow. It is possible that evaluation of prostatic tumor cell populations by flow cytometry or perhaps relative nuclear roundness factor may provide a more accurate predictor of growth rate.

2. Metastatic Potential

With few exceptions, prostatic cancer **mortality is related to metastasis**. Most prostatic cancers seem to have the ability to metastasize, but both autopsy and clinical experiences suggest that this capacity may be lacking in some.

a) **Metastatic potential is currently assessed by clinical staging**. Refinements in clinical staging techniques have contributed to the continuous improvement in survival rates of patients variously treated for apparently localized tumors by excluding those lesions recognized to have already metastasized.

b) **Pelvic lymph node dissection is one of the more important staging procedures.** It has led to the discovery of clinically unsuspected regional lymph node metastases in a significant proportion of patients with stage T2 prostatic cancer. The frequency of nodal metastasis increases with increasing volume of local disease as reflected in the subcategories of stage T2 tumors.

Regional lymph node metastasis may be the first and only site of clinically detectable metastasis in patients otherwise selected to be free of spread of prostatic cancer.

Regional lymph node metastasis should be regarded as an indication of disseminated disease: more than 75% of patients with demonstrable lymph node metastasis will develop clinical evidence of other metastatic tumor within 5 years

c) **In conclusion.** In practical terms the metastatic potential of a prostatic cancer is positively indicated only by the identification of metastases, and clinical staging techniques and staging lymphadenectomy are the measures employed to assess this potential. Another important consideration is that recognized regional metastasis represents the biological potential of a given neoplasm at only one particular point in time. A small localized tumor may in fact have already been inherently programmed to metastasize regardless of therapy. This is a sobering and pessimistic possibility, but one that is not inconsistent with the uncertainties regarding metastatic potential of a particular neoplasm as well as assessments of the end results of treatment.

3. Stage Progression

a) Both **growth rate** and **metastatic potential** determine the pattern of stage progression of a prostatic cancer.

The sequence T1 → T2 → T3-4 → N+/ M+ is a simple and logical possibility but one that epitomizes only a portion of the stage progression spectrum. All other possibilities of stage progression can and do occur. With regard to a stage T2 cancer, it may remain localized as such throughout the lifetime of the host, it may manifest focal growth and local invasion and progress directly to a stage T3, or it may "silently" invade lymphatics and/or the bloodstream to disseminate, implant successfully, and develop metastatic growth recognized as stage N+ / M+ disease, without exhibiting local growth sufficient to permit its prior detection as a stage T3 lesion. **The younger the patient** with stage T2 cancer at the time of diagnosis, **the greater the probability that the cancer will metastasize** and adversely affect life expectancy.

b) **The earlier the stage** of the tumor at diagnosis, **the greater the possible patterns of tumor behavior**, the larger the number of therapeutic options, and the greater the difficulty in evaluating the impact of the therapy upon the subsequent clinical course.

4. Conclusion

From the urologist's standpoint, one may summarize current conceptions of the natural history of stage T2 prostatic cancers by saying that both **growth rate** and **metastatic potential** are important determinants of stage progression and of the end results of therapy, that these variables can currently be determined only by serial observations over time, that the urologist has no certain and practical way of predicting the course of disease at the time of his initial contact with the patient, and that he is therefore disadvantaged in projecting the need for "optimal" treatment and in evaluating the results of his treatment.

III. MANAGEMENT OF STAGE T2 PROSTATIC CANCER

General considerations

Although the actual or potential biological activity of stage T2 prostatic cancer cannot be established with certainty, the fact that lethal carcinomas are currently indistinguishable from those that are not, generally persuades the clinician to recommend some form of treatment, an approach which is also often demanded by the patient.

The options of therapy for stage T2 tumors include:

1) Observation only (with treatment at first evidence of disease progression),

2) Radical prostatectomy (perineal or retropubic, with or without regional lymph node dissection), or

3) Radiation therapy (megavoltage external beam or interstitial irradiation with either I-125 or gold-198, with or without pelvic lymph node dissection), and

4) Modifications or **combinations** of the aforementioned therapies.

◆ **Objectives of the radical treatment** (surgery or radiotherapy): To cure prostatic cancer with surgery, all tumor must be excised. To cure prostatic cancer with irradiation, all tumor cells must be destroyed, or at least their growth rate must be sufficiently arrested to permit the cancer to be contained within the prostate for years (long enough for the patient to die of another cause). Success of both "curative" therapies is measured in time.

1. No treatment option

In an individual 65-70 years or older, or with an anticipated life expectancy of 5 years or less, observation only may be the preferred and most appropriate management for a stage T2 cancer since its rate of growth may be quite slow.

Experience at MSKCC and the results of the VACURG study have shown that some localized prostatic tumors may not progress, or do so so slowly within the finite lifetime of the host that they do not require treatment, whereas some patients may indeed benefit from radical prostatectomy, and many tumors destined to progress may have already done so by the time treatment was begun.

The challenge is then to identify and select:

a) Those tumors that need radical excision (or radiation therapy) to ensure adequate control and long-term survival, and

b) Those tumors **not destined to progress** and threaten the life of the patient, which need no immediate treatment.

The no treatment option is a balanced decision between how long the patient is expected to live normally and how soon the cancer may be expected to express its potential clinical morbidity (at age 63, 10-year expected survival is 64% based upon life-table analysis).

Table 1. Survival after various treatments for stage B (T2) prostatic cancer

Treatment	Author	Stage	No. patients (years)	Survival (% patients alive)		
				5 years	10 years	15 years
RP	Jewett [2]	B_1	103 (1909-51)	–	50	27
		B_2	79 (1909-51)	–	41	18
RP	Walsh and Jewett [2]	B_1	57 (1951-63)	~ 93	~ 70	51
		B_2	53 (1951-63)	~ 75	~ 50	~ 25
ERT	Bagshaw [11]	B	426 (1956-80)	79	58	37
		B_1	35	~ 86	~ 82	~ 82
		B_2	113	~ 86	~ 70	~ 56
I-125	Whitmore [12]	B_1	24 (1970-85)	84	58 (54 %)	–
		B_2	52 (1970-85)	92	62 (23 %)	–
		B_3	23 (1970-85)	66	15 (13 %)	–
Au-198 and ERT	Scardino [13]	B_{1a}	26 (1965-79)	93 (94 %)	82 (71 %)	–
		B_1	94	86 (61 %)	71 (–)	–
		B_2	110	90 (69 %)	82 (57 %)	–

RP = radical prostatectomy; ERT = external radiation therapy; % patients alive in RP series = disease-free survival; ~ = approximations from survival curves; ( ) = disease-free survival in ERT and interstitial irradiation series.

2. Radical prostatectomy versus radiation therapy for stage T2 disease

Survival after various treatments for stage T2 prostatic cancer is shown in Table 1. These include experiences with radical prostatectomy, external beam irradiation, and two methods of interstitial irradiation I-125 implantation and combined interstitial (gold-198) and external irradiation. Pathologic stage of disease is given for the radical surgery series and the percentage of patients alive represents clinical disease-free survival.

a) Radical prostatectomy

Radical prostatectomy is associated with impressive long-term, disease-free survival in a significant number of patients with stage T2 tumors.

However, in the original Johns Hopkins (JH) series, 37% of the 103 patients with 1.5 cm nodules (stage T2a) ultimately died of carcinoma of the prostate, and the deaths occurred at a steady rate up to 15 years of follow-up. Another 36% died before 15 years of follow-up of causes unrelated to prostatic cancer.

In stageT2b (B2) disease, 18% of the total B2 group were alive and tumor-free at 15 years. Somewhat better survival results are presented in the later JH series, but 13 patients lost to follow-up are excluded, and the overall results in patients pathologically staged are not so much better than can be accounted for by differences in case selection. Nevertheless, it is difficult to escape the conclusion that *some patients with localized prostatic cancers are probably alive because of their radical prostatectomy*, although the overall impact of radical surgery with regard to the total JH experience of 3,711 patients (1909-1966) has resulted in no more than 1-2% of all patients with prostatic cancer being cured of their disease.

Such statistics, however, ignore the population at risk from whom patients were selected for radical surgery, and they generally have little impact in considering management of individual patients.

b) Radiotherapy

Megavoltage external beam irradiation *may achieve comparable survival results to radical prostatectomy*, but such patients are alive both with and without disease, and the survival figures are actuarial or projected since fewer patients have actually been at risk or followed for up to 15 years. However, it should be noted that of the 37% 15-year survival reported from Stanford, only 6% of patients had T2a disease; that is, 94% of these radiated patients had more advanced disease than those included in the radical prostatectomy series.

Meaningful survival data beyond 10 years are not yet available for any form of interstitial irradiation. Schellhammer has recently updated his results with I-125 irradiation. Actuarial disease-free survival at 5 and 7 years is 100% for stage T2a disease (17 patients), and absolute survival at 5 years (6 patients) is also 100%.

For T2b lesions, actuarial survival is 73% at 5 and 7 years, and 80% (23 cases) absolute survival at 5 years after treatment. These results are somewhat better than at MSKCC.

The **overall results of different methods** of treatment for apparently localized stage T2 prostatic cancer **reveal a remarkable similarity in the 5-, 10-, and 15** (where available) **year survival rates** both with and without disease. However, one must acknowledge that such data are assembled from different institutions, at different times, and using different staging criteria, different selection criteria (more stringent in later years), different means of calculating survival results, and, most importantly, different criteria for determining freedom of evidence of neoplasm.

c) **Is there contemporary evidence to suggest whether radical surgery or radiation therapy is superior in producing disease-free survival in patients with localized prostatic cancer ?**

1. *Studies comparing occurrence of metastases*

◆ *Uro-Oncology Research Group study* The Uro-Oncology Research Group re-

cently compared megavoltage radiotherapy versus radical prostatectomy in a randomized clinical trial for patients with stage T2 prostatic cancer.

Treatment failure occurred in 4 (10%) of 41 patients allocated to receive radical surgery. Of the 56 patients treated with radiation therapy, 17 (30%) relapsed . This study suggests that a radical operation is more effective than megavoltage irradiation in controlling prostatic cancer. Local recurrence was not addressed in the randomized study, so the true impact of these two forms of localized therapy cannot be evaluated with certainty.

◆ *Olsson et al.* : 69 patients with surgically staged T1 b and T2 adenocarcinoma of the prostate were managed by radical prostatectomy (37 patients), I-125 implantations (25 patients) or external beam irradiation (7 patients).

Analysis of the 3 treatments by Kaplan-Meier technique revealed nearly identical distant failure curves for radical prostatectomy and interstitial irradiation (8.1% and 8.0%, respectively), with both demonstrating a near significant advantage comparative to external radiotherapy (28.6%)

2. *Studies comparing local recurrences*

Table II shows treatment failures after various forms of irradiation or radical prostatectomy. Such data must be considered with caution, however, since the frequency of local recurrences after radical prostatectomy is often not determined or poorly documented, and the definition of local control in the radiation series is clinically and not often pathologically determined . Despite such qualifications, the local recurrence rate alone is remarkably similar after either radical surgery or radiotherapy, both megavoltage and interstitial irradiation (Belt and Schroeder, Culp).

Table 2. Treatment failure after various treatments for stage B (T2) prostatic cancer

Treatment	Author	Stage	No. patients	LR (%)	DM (%)	LR & DM (%)
RP	Jewett [14]	B₁(P)	86	6 (7)	7 (8)	8 (9)
RP	Culp [15]	B₁	123	19 (15)	10 (8)	14 (11)
RP	Belt [16]	B,C	464	79 (17)	61 (13)	–
		B(P)	185	59 (22)	50 (19)	–
		C(P)	266	59 (22)	50 (19)	–
ERT	Bagshaw [11]	B,C	1,114	145 (13)	256 (23)	–
I-125	Whitmore [1, 17]	B,C	589	57 (9)	169 (30)	–
		B₁	340	20 (6)	53 (16)	–
		B₂	123	14 (11)	51 (40)	–
		B₃,C	126	23 (18)	65 (52)	–

ᵃ(P) = pathological stage of disease; LR = local recurrence alone; DM = distant metastases.

3) *Meaning of post-irradiation biopsy*

A biopsy suggesting residual viable tumor cells 1-2.5 years after completion of radiation therapy may indicate a radioresistant tumor and ultimately predict treatment failure. However, whether this may herald early metastatic disease, local recurrence, or both, remains to be clarified. Stated another way, failure to respond to irradiation, as determined by biopsy, may simply identify a more virulent cancer that has already metastasized at the time of local treatment.

3. Conclusion

Accepting the overall similarity in at least 10-year-survival rates, and comparable local control rates, in patients with stage T2 prostatic cancer receiving no treatment, various forms of irradiation, or radical excision, one may conclude, as an **optimist**, that a variety of treatments offer similar prospects of benefit, or, as a **pessimist**, that none of the treatments is producing a significant beneficial effect and that the survivals are a consequence of the natural history of the disease.

A possibility that has yet to be evaluated, however, is that different treatments produce benefit in different segments of the stage T2 prostatic cancer population: it supports the possibility that within a given tumor there may exist populations of cells responsive or unresponsive to irradiation,

chemotherapy, and endocrine therapy, and that appropriate combinations of treatments may succeed in eradicating a tumor in a setting where a single treatment would be certain to fail. The challenge also is to identify those early localized and confined prostatic cancers that will not respond to irradiation or other forms of treatment, and whose biological potential can be functionally characterized as aggressive tumors destined to spread but that have not yet done so at the time of evaluation. Such tumors may be excised before they metastasize and threaten both the quality and quantity of life of the patient.

This is no mean task for future research, but one that offers the possibility of improved understanding of the biology of localized prostatic cancer, and thereby of more appropriate and effective therapy, rather than engaging in continued polemics regarding which form of therapy is preferred for all patients afflicted with such an unpredictable and heterogeneous tumor as prostatic cancer. The long-term goal remains the identification of the best method of treatment for the individual patient, whatever that method proves to be.

IV. WHAT TREATMENT FOR WHICH PATIENT?

While different treatment methods yield comparable overall 10-15 years survival results, a definitive therapeutic decision can be made relative to differences in local control and quality of life. The choice of therapy, therefore is based on 2 main considerations: **tumor control** and **host**.

On the basis of tumor control alone, treatment selection can be segregated in 3 age categories.

• In **young patients** (40-60 years of age), radical prostatectomy provides the best chances of durable disease-free survival.

• In **patients between 60 and 70 years of age**, radical prostatectomy and radiation therapy (external or interstitial) achieve similar degree of tumor control and both options can be offered as adequate alternative therapies.

• **Above 70 years of age**, radiation therapy or observation only (therapy deferred until objective progression occurs) offer similar satisfactory tumor control.

• Within each age category, the selection of therapy must take into account factors such as quality of life (sexual potency, stress incontinence, etc..), potential complications from therapy and the presence of medical problems that may increase the risks of therapy or reduce significantly the patient's life expectancy.

DOCUMENTATION

BAGSHAW MA: External beam radiation therapy of prostatic carcinoma. AUA Videoconf Prostatic Cancer 15-22, 1982.

BELT E, SCHROEDER FH: Total perineal prostatectomy for carcinoma of the prostate. J Urol 107: 91-96,1972.

BYAR DP, CORLE DK: VACURG randomized trial of radical prostatectomy for stage 1 and 2 prostate cancer, Urology 1 7:7-1 1, 1 981 .

CULPOS: Radical perineal prostatectomy: Its past, present and possible future. J. Urol 1 07:91 -96,1 972.

DIAMOND DA, BERRY SJ, UMBRICHT C, JEWETT JH,

COFFEY DS: Computerized image analysis of nuclear shape as a prognostic factor for prostatic cancer. The prostate 3:321-332,1982.

FIDLER IJ: Tumor heterogeneity and the biology of cancer invasion and metastasis. Cancer Res 38:2651-2660,1980.

FOWLER JE Jr, WHITMORE WF Jr : The incidence and extent of pelvic lymph node metastases in apparently localized prostatic cancer. Cancer 47: 2945-2945, 1981.

JEWETT HJ: The present status of radical prostatectomy for stage A and B prostatic cancer. Urol Clin North Am 2 : 105-124, 1975.

MADOR D, RITCHIE B, MEEKER B, MOORE R, EL-LIOTT FG, McPHEE MS, CHAPMAN JD, LAKEY WH: Response of the Dunning R 3327H prostatic adenocarcinoma to radiation and various chemotherapeutic drugs. Cancer Treat Rep 66 :1 837-1 843,1 982.

OLSSON C.A: Surgical management of stage T2 or C prostatic carcinoma: radical surgery vs radiotherapy. Supplement to   Urology, 25: 30,1985.

PAULSON DF, LIN GH, INSHAW W, STEPHANI S: The Uro-Oncology Research Group. Radical surgery versus radiotherapy for adenocarcinoma of the prostate. J Urol 128: 502-504.

RONSTROM L, TRIBUKAIT B, ESPOSTI PL: DNA pattern and cytological findings in fine-needle aspirates of untreated prostatic tumors. A flow cytofluorometric study. The prostate 2: 79-88, 1981.

ROSENBERG S., WHITMORE W.F: Delayed treatment of adenocarcinoma of the prostate. MSKCC Urologic tumor symposium, 1984.

SCARDINO PT: Combined interstitial (gold 198) and external for localized prostatic cancer. AUA Videoconf Prostatic Cancer 136-142, 1 982.

SCHELHAMMER PF: Personal communication.

STAMEY TA: Cancer of the prostate, Monogr Urol 3:67-94, 1982.

SUFFRIN G: Personal communication.

WALSH PC, Jewett, HJ: Radical surgery for prostatic cancer. Cancer 45: 1906-1911, 1980.

WHITMORE WF Jr: Interstitial radiation therapy for carcinoma of the prostate. The prostate 1 :157-168,1980.

WHITMORE W.F et al: I-125 implantation for carcinoma of the prostate.

WHITMORE W.F Jr, HILARIS B: Personal communication.

III

MANAGEMENT OF FAILURES AFTER RADICAL TREATMENT FOR LOCALIZED DISEASE

Prostate Specific Antigen for Early Detection of Recurrences after Surgery

Paul H. Lange.

Department of Urology, University of Washington Medical Center, Seattle, Washington.

Much has been written suggesting that Prostate Specific Antigen (PSA) is a useful, if not indispensable, serum tumor marker for a variety of clinical situations related to carcinoma of the prostate. We will concentrate in this presentation on the value of serum PSA levels after radical prostatectomy in predicting persistent disease and the response to adjuvant therapies.

I. SERUM PSA LEVELS.

Perhaps the most exciting use of PSA is in **determining residual disease after radical prostatectomy**. In theory, no PSA should be present within the circulation if **all prostatic tissue** (benign and malignant) has been removed. In practice, this application is limited by the sensitivity and precision of the PSA assays.

The exact level of PSA that can confidently be assumed to represent **actual PSA within the circulation varies between assays and, most importantly, within each laboratory** for a given assay.

In general, about 20% to 25% of patients have elevated PSA levels an average of 1 to 2 years **after surgery**, and the prevalence of these elevations increases with pathologic stage (Table 1).

We analyzed the value of PSA levels 3 to 6 months after radical prostatectomy using a value of 0.4 ng/ml (Tandem® assay) as the lower limit of detectability (Table 2) .

◆ **1)** Among men whose PSA was **less than 0.2 ng/ml, only 11 % demonstrated recurrence** as evidenced by the development of a positive bone scan or progressively elevated PSA levels within 6 to 50 months.

◆ **2)** In contrast, in men whose 3- to 6-month PSA level was **0.4 ng/ml or higher**, there was evidence of **recurrence in 100 %** during a follow-up ranging from 7 to 75 months.

◆ **3)** We also analyzed the **pathologic stages** of the disease in patients whose PSA was known after radical prostatectomy. In general, **95% of the patients with eleva-**

Table 1. Frequency of elevated PSA levels after radical prostatectomy .

MEAN FOLLOW-UP (MONTHS) (SD)	NUMBER OF PATIENTS/TOTAL (%)			TOTAL (%)
	OC	CP Only	+SV/+LN	
21.7 (15.3)	7/71 (10)	5/23 (22)	16/22 (73)	24
24	2/81 (20)	5/20 (25)	20/26 (77)	21
12			13/21 (62)	

OC = organ-confined disease; CP = capsular perforation with or without positive margin; +SV = positive seminal vesicles; +LN = positive seminal vesicles; +N = positive lymph nodes.

Table 2. Serum PSA levels (ng/ml) 3 to 6 months after radical prostatectomy and clinical outcome.

	<0.2	>0.4	0.3
No.	35	16	5
Recurrence (%)	3 (11)	16 (100)	3 (60)
Follow-up: mean (range)	25 (6–71)	17 (7–75)	17 (6–28)

Data from Lightner DJ, Lange PH, Reddy PK, et al: PSA and local recurrence after radical prostatectomy. J Urol (in press)

ted PSA concentrations 3 to 6 months after radical prostatectomy were **high risk patients** who had positive margins, seminal vesicles, or lymph nodes involvement.

◆ **4)** However, **among all the high-risk** pathologic groups, PSA was **undetectable** (below 0.2 ng/ml) **in 37 %.** Thus it may be that:

• **initially abnormal PSA levels** merely identify those high-risk patients whose disease is **destined to recur early** and that

• among patients whose postoperative **PSA value is below 0.2 ng/ml, more recurrences will be detected with longer follow-up.**

In our experience, all of those patients whose disease recurred had elevated PSAs before the recurrence, although undoubtedly, there will be exceptions to this rule.

Thus the value of post prostatectomy PSA is initially normal in a significant number of patients after radical prostatectomy who **subsequently develop elevated PSA levels and then recurrence.** This may be because the volume of residual disease is not sufficient to raise the systemic PSA level, or the production of PSA by the residual tumor cells may be suppressed. Either circumstance suggests future strategies for enhancing the value of postoperative PSA. For example, more sensitive PSA assays could be developed: **ultrasensitive PSA** measurement is one of the possible ways to achieve this **very early detection of recurrences.**

II. ORIGIN OF PSA ELEVATION.

Determining the **location of disease** in patients with **unequivocal elevations in PSA after radical prostatectomy** is a problem which is getting increasing attention.

1. Local recurrence or metastasis?

a) We studied 63 patients whose PSA was **elevated** 6 to 240 months **after radical prostatectomy** and who had no other treatment.

• In 6, **metastasis** was found by prostatic acid phosphatase levels, cystoscopy, bone scan, or CT of the abdomen.

• However, in 57 men, these **studies were negative.**

Yet we found that when a **needle biopsy** of the urethrovesical anastomotic area was performed, about **40% were positive** for prostate adenocarcinoma.

b) Furthermore, in 30 men whose **PSA was normal, none had a positive anastomotic biopsy.**

Surprisingly, the **rectal examination** was not significantly different between those patients with and without a positive anastomotic biopsy or between those patients with and without an elevated PSA level.

These results suggest that **PSA is an excellent indicator of possible persistent local disease after radical prostatectomy.** Local recurrence with a normal PSA has been reported, but it is exceedingly rare. Moreover, at least at an early stage, **rectal examination does not seem to discriminate well between patients with and without local disease.**

2. Incidence of localized disease:

Does this unexpected high percentage of persistent disease mean that local disease is **more common than heretofore realized?**

The answer is unknown, but intelligent speculation is possible.

◆ For example, the local disease occurred in only about 40% of a non consecutive group of patients with elevated PSA concentrations and not in any of the patients with normal levels.

As previously discussed, the approximate frequency of elevated PSA concentrations among patients who have had radical prostatectomy is still incompletely known but so far has averaged 20% to 25%.

A worst case scenario would be that all patients whose disease recur after radical prostatectomy have elevated PSA conentrations and that 50% ultimately fail. In this case, the percentage of positive anastomotic biopsies would be 20% (=50% recurrence times 40% positive biopsies). Such a figure is within the range of local recurrence seen in some series with longer follow-ups.

Thus, *PSA and early anastomotic biopsy* may merely *pick up disease later recognized by more classic methods*.

◆ Alternatively, a 20% prevalence of local recurrence may mean that *local disease is more common than heretofore appreciated*, because the figure is higher than in some series with longer follow-ups. Thus, the true instance of local disease in patients with an elevated PSA concentration may be greater than our 40% figure because undoubtedly, some sampling error occurs with the anastomotic biopsy.

The fact remains that the worst-case scenario is that PSA and anastomotic biopsies are detecting a prevalence of local recurrence after radical prostatectomy that is only twice as great as heretofore appreciated.

3. Response of PSA levels to radiation therapy:

The response of patients to radiation therapy after radical prostatectomy also contributes information about the location of disease in patients whose PSA is elevated.

In those patients whose PSA is definitely elevated after radical prostatectomy, adjuvant *radiation therapy causes the PSA to decrease by 80% and to undetectable levels in 53%,* even in some patients who are biopsy negative. In stage N+ disease, PSA was reduced by 50 % in eight of nine patients and to female levels in four.

III. TIME COURSE OF PSA LEVELS AND RECURRENCE

The durability of suppressed PSA levels after radiation therapy given either as adjuvant or as active treatment because of an elevated PSA is unknown. Certainly, patients whose PSA *decreased by 50 %* but not to undetectable levels seemed to obtain *little therapeutic effect*. In addition, in our retrospective series, only about half the patients whose serum PSA became **undetectable after radiation therapy** have sustained an undetectable level after 20 months. It is impossible to determine whether this re-elevation of PSA levels is attributable to regrowth or persistent regional disease after radiation therapy or to further growth of existing distant metastases. It would not be surprising that the radiation therapy given in these patients would not permanently sterilize locoregional disease in most patients.

Whether radiation therapy will nonetheless prolong survival is also unknown.

IV. CONCLUSION.

Despite these therapeutic uncertainties, our data suggest that after radical prostatectomy, *persistent locoregional disease is the predominant, and possibly the only, residual disease in some patients who ultimately fail.*

If this is true, **new therapies** should be tested such as more extensive surgical excision or better radiotherapy.

What is undeniable now is that investigations of patients with elevated PSA levels after radical prostatectomy will **increase our understanding** of persistent disease after radical prostatectomy.

DOCUMENTATION

BRAWER MK, LANGE PH: PSA in the screening, staging and followup of early state prostate cancer: A review of recent developments. World J Uro 3:227,1989

ERCOLE CJ, LANGE PH, MATHISEN M, et al: Prostatic specific antigen and prostatic acid phosphatase in the monitoring and staging of patients with prostatic cancer. J Urol I38 :1181, I987

HUDSON MA, BAHNSON RB, CATALONA WJ: Clinical use of prostate specific antigen in patients with prostate cancer. J Urol I42 :10ll, 1989

LANGE PH, ERCOLE CJ, LIGHTNER DJ, et al: Value of serum prostatic specific antigen determinations before and after radical prostatectomy. J Urol,141:873,1989

OESTERLING JE, CHAN DW, EPSTEIN JI, et al: Prostate specific antigen in the preoperative and post-operative evaluation of localized prostatic cancer treated with radical prostatectomy. J Urol, 139:766,1988

STAMEY TA, KABALIN JN, MCNEAL JE, et al: Prostatic specific antigen in the diagnosis and treatment of adenocarcinoma of the prostate II: Radical prostatectomy treated patients. J Urol, I41, I076,1989

Can the failure of radiotherapy be predicted by the post-treatment PSA level ?

K.J. Russell et al.
J. Urol. 146, 1046 (1991)

Although the variations in PSA levels are well known after radical prostatectomy, little data is available concerning the course of PSA after radiotherapy. We reviewed the records of patients treated at 5 external beam radiotherapy institutions in the greater Seattle metropolitan area in order to analyse the possible relationship between variations in PSA and the clinical course after radiotherapy and to measure the role of PSA in the early detection of cancer recurrence.

143 patients with stage A1 to D1 disease had received radiotherapy with curative intent and were followed for an average of 27 months or until recurrence. Response to treatment was classified into the following three categories : 1) complete response, 2) clinical failure defined by the discovery of recurrence either on digital rectal examination or on bone scan or any other imaging modality or by biopsy, but only counted chronologically from the date at which symptoms justified hormonal manipulation, 3) chemical failure, corresponding to an isolated rise in PSA to above the normal limits of the laboratory.

Conclusion 1 : As expected, there was a significant *correlation between the stage and the complete response rate :* the higher the PSA, the lower the chance of remaining in complete response.

Conclusion 2 : In 59 cases, a PSA level was available 6 months after completion of radiotherapy. Of the 34 patients in whom PSA returned to normal over 6 months, 32 (94%) remained in complete remission versus only 2 (8%) with progression (p = 0.0001) . However, 24 of these complete responder patients with a normal PSA at 6 months had a pretreatment PSA of 2.1 times normal, while the others had a PSA of 35.4 times normal. Patients with low stage and grade tumours had a greater than 90% probability of having a normal PSA level within 6 months of treatment. PSA values 12 months after treatment were available in 85 patients = normalization of PSA was again found to be correlated with a significantly higher success rate : only 7% of clinical failures versus 61% when PSA had not returned to normal after one year. The favourable significance of normalization of PSA at 6 or 12 months after treatment is therefore the major contribution of this marker in the follow-up of the course of irradiated prostatic cancer. When PSA returns to normal, it does so within 6 to 12 months in 90% of cases. It is too early to predict how long patients in whom PSA returns to normal and who respond to radiotherapy will stay in remission. *However, it is already clear that those patients in whom PSA either fails to return to normal or rises have a very poor prognosis.*

Conclusion 3 : 23 *biopsies* were performed and, in 19 cases, these patients had a PSA assay within 3 months of the procedure. 72% of patients with a positive biopsy had elevated PSA values versus 20% with a negative biopsy. 91% of patients with elevated PSA (versus 50% with normal PSA) had a positive biopsy.

Conclusion 4 : When PSA was elevated, it was very rare (8%) that it did not continue to increase gradually, thereby eliminating any possible doubt about an initial minor elevation.

Conclusion 5 : Patients with a *high initial PSA* (more than 4 times normal) had a lower probability (43%) of responding than when the PSA was < 4 times normal (83%).

Conclusion 6 : It would appear reasonable to propose alternative treatment protocols for patients in whom *PSA does not return to normal within 1 year.*

Local Failure After Definitive Treatment of Carcinoma of the Prostate

Paul F. Schellhammer and Anas M .El-Mahdi

Department of Urology and Radiation Oncology, Eastern Virginia Medical School, Norfolk, Virginia. USA

The present discussion is directed at the issue of *failure of definitive therapy to achieve tumor control* and the *distant dissemination and local morbidity associated with local failure*. It is based on the experience at Eastern Virginia Medical School (EVMS) with 118 patients treated by I-125 implantation, 317 patients treated by external-beam irradiation and 67 patients treated by radical prostatectomy. One hundred and eight of the first group, 178 of the second, and all of the third have been followed 8 or more years after treatment.

Local control of cancer is the primary expectation of a locally directed therapy, and the success in achieving lasting local control is a good measure of the treatment's efficacy.

I. CAUSES OF LOCAL FAILURE

After radical prostatectomy, local failure most likely reflects incomplete resection of tumor cells.

After radiation therapy, the situation is more complex.

Failure may result from clones of cells totally resistant to radiation or of cells that undergo sublethal damage and are able, subsequently, to recover and resume growth. It may also result from the development of new tumors in an organ at risk left in situ. In addition, inadequate external-beam treatment portals may result in radiologic "misses" so that cells outside the field are untreated and subsequently cause local failure. This is especially a problem in the treatment of clinical stage T3 cancer. Because any one of the above factors may give rise to local failure, there is a significant potential for local failure after definitive irradiation.

II. CLINICAL DATA

1. Biopsy Data

a) After radiotherapy

Our results showed that patients with a *positive biopsy* 18 or more months after I-125 implantation or external beam irradiation subsequently demonstrated a statistically higher incidence of *both local and distant failure* than patients with negative biopsies. Within pretreatment stage and grade subcategories, positive biopsy remained a statistically significant predictor of subsequent failure with either modality of therapy. However, at a median of 11 years, 4 of 22 (18%) biopsy-positive patients remain without clinical evidence of disease.

Currently, we do not routinely perform prostate biopsy after irradiation but *restrict the procedure to patients who develop an abnormal prostate examination* and for whom *hormonal or surgical therapy would be appropriate* (as determined by stage, grade, age, general health, and interval to failure) if the biopsy were positive.

b) After radical surgery

A positive surgical margin after radical prostatectomy or a postsurgical biopsy positive for residual neoplasm at the clinically normal urethrovesical anastomosis would appear to carry the same adverse implications as a positive biopsy from a palpably normal prostate after irradiation. Lange and colleagues performed blind needle biopsy of the bladder neck anastomosis in men with detectable prostate-specific antigen levels but without palpable abnormalities after radical prostatectomy. In 39%, the biopsy was positive for adenocarcinoma. Positive surgical margins have been found in 18% to 50% of clinical stage T2 tumors. Therefore, *persistent local disease after radical prostatectomy is not uncommon*. Its true incidence, natural history, and eventual clinical impact have become subjects of scrutiny.

2. Interpretation of Clinical Data

Follow-up beyond 5 years is necessary to document local failure accurately.

12% of local failures in our series, 15 % of those in Culp's series, and 28 % of those in the series of Blute and coworkers occurred 10 or more years after surgery.

The reported incidence of local failure represents the minimum, as patients who have distant failure may have local failure masked by hormonal therapy or may die of cancer or unrelated causes prior to clinical local recurrence.

a) Local Failure After Irradiation

Our initial study of local tumor recurrence among patients managed with I-125 and followed for at least 5 years showed a progressive increase in the local failure rate with increasing T stage and lesser degrees of tumor differentiation.

The failure of I-125 to maintain local control over time is evidenced by the fact that more than 50% of our local failures occurred after 5 years.

Local failure rates in those few irradiation series not employing concomitant hormone therapy are listed in Table 1.

b) Local Failure After Radical Prostatectomy

Observations regarding local failure after surgery were first made by Whitmore in 1959, and the question was re-examined 10 years later by Jewett and coworkers. Two decades later, information concerning local failure according to clinical and pathologic stage after unaided radical prostatectomy with follow-up of 5, 10, and 15 years remains limited.

Table 1. Local failure by clinical stage after external-beam radiation without hormonal therapy

	A		B		C		
	No.	(%)	No.	(%)	No.	(%)	FOLLOW-UP (YEARS)
Gibbons et al[29]	–		–		17/209	(8)	>2
Neglia et al[71]	–		0/3	(0)	7/76	(9)	2–8
EVMS series	2/43	(4.6)	4/24	(17)	42/150	(28)	5–10
			20/100†	(20)			

*Stage B1N.
†Stage B2.

Table 2. Local failure by clinical stage after radical prostatectomy *

	A2		B		C		
	No.	*(%)*	*No.*	*(%)*	*No.*	*(%)*	FOLLOW-UP (YEARS)
Nichols et al[72]	3/33	(10)	–	–	–	–	10
Middleton et al[65]	2/40	(5)	–	–	–	–	5
Culp[16]	–	–	33/123	(26)	–	–	1–15
Gibbons et al[28]	–	–	5/52	(10)	–	–	15
Middleton et al[65]	–	–	–	(28)	–	–	10
Zincke et al[105]	–	–	–	–	13/47	(28)	1–17
Walsh and Jewett[100]	–	–	7/57	(12)	–	–	15
Schellhammer[88]	–	–	4/26	(15)	3/4	(75)	15
Total	5/77	(6)	49/258	(19)	16/51	(31)	

*No hormone therapy used in these series.

• **Clinical Stage T1b.** Middleton and associates reported local failure in 2 of 40 (5 %) and Nichols and coworkers in 3 of 33 (9 %) patients followed through 5 years (Table 6).

• *Clinical Stage T2.* : The local failure rate for stage **T2a** is around 5% at 5 years and 10% at 15 years; for stage **T2b**, it was 12% at 5 years and 16% at 15 years. However, Culp reported a 26% local failure rate at 1 to 15 years in T1a lesions.

Pathologic Stage T2 : The landmark series of Jewett and associates reported a 16% local failure rate at 15 years. In our series, the local failure at 15 years was 17%.

• *Clinical Stage T3 :* Few series have reported local failure rates after surgical excision of clinical stage T3 disease. Zincke and coworkers found local failure in 28% after unaided radical prostatectomy for stage T3. McCullough and Leadbetter reported a 50%, and Spaulding and Whitmore a 52%, local failure rate after extended surgical excision.

Pathologic Stage T3: Pathologic stage T3 describes a wide spectrum of histologic findings; extracapsular disease and seminal vesicle involvement are universally accepted criteria for stage T3 disease, but capsule involvement and extent (penetration versus perforation) have not been clearly characterized in all series. The local failure rate at 15 years in our series using the criteria of extracapsular disease or seminal vesicle invasion was 31%

which is in agreement with that of other large series.

In our series, of the nine patients with a positive seminal vesicle, local failure occurred in four (44%). In contrast, the Mayo Clinic did not find seminal vesicle invasion to be associated with an adverse prognosis.

• *Stage N+:* The incidence of local failure for node positive patients has infrequently been analysed separately. Zinke noted a 25% failure rate at 10 years, which is much less than our 50% failure rate after implantation of I-125, irrespective of the T stage of the primary tumor.

III. TREATMENT OF LOCAL FAILURE

The treatment of local failure is identified as adjunctive or *prophylactic* when administered to patients at high risk for local failure namely those patients whose tumors clinically or histologically demonstrate capsule perforation or positive margins or seminal vesicles and who have a detectable or elevated prostate-specific antigen level. Treatment is identified as *therapeutic* when administered to patients in whom local failure already has occurred.

1. Prophylactic Therapy

• *Clinical Stage T2.* Carson reported the Mayo Clinic experience with radical retropubic prostatectomy and pelvic lymphadenectomy

4 to 8 weeks after planned preoperative external-beam radiotherapy in nine patients. Follow-up ranged from 18 months to 11 years, during which time three patients had metastatic disease. The postoperative morbidity was not affected by the radiation therapy.

• *Clinical Stage T3.* Spaulding and Whitmore and McCullough and Leadbetter demonstrated that **extended excision** can be performed with acceptable morbidity in patients with clinical evidence of locally advanced disease. They suggested that it be used only after other therapeutic options were exhausted. The local failure rate after a surgical attempt to treat clinical stage T3 tumors is high: 41 to 52%.

The first use of **adjunctive irradiation** was reported by Flocks and coworkers, who injected a colloidal suspension of 100 mCi of Au-198 into the resection margins after radical prostatectomy for clinical stage T3 prostate cancer. Local recurrence was detected in only 3 (4.5 per cent) after a 15 year follow up.

Pathologic Stage T3. A number of series have reported the use of *prophylactic postoperative external-beam radiation after radical prostatectomy in patients with histologic extracapsular tumor excision.* Comparative assessment is difficult because of the already mentioned wide spectrum of disease included in the definition of pathologic stage T3 and the variability in radiation dose field size and in follow-up. With short follow-up, Forman and Pilepich and their associates reported complete local tumor control and few complications among patients treated with postprostatectomy irradiation. Ray and coworkers used 70 Gy in patients with capsular penetration, seminal vesicle invasion, or invasion of the bladder neck. The treatment was well tolerated. Local control was achieved in 77% with follow-up extending to 10 years.

In the series of Lange and coworkers, the largest and most thoroughly studied postoperative irradiation experience, 35 patients with positive surgical margins or seminal vesicle invasion were treated. Only three (10%) of the patients experienced complications beyond 6 months. Modified lymphadenectomy, limitation of radiation to 60 Gy to the pelvis, and treatment after **complete recovery from surgery** contributed to the low morbidity. *After a 2.5- to 10-year follow-up, only 1 of 35 (3%) of the patients had manifested a local recurrence.*

On the other hand, Paulson compared the probabilities of failure and survival in 63 patients with T3 disease who had surgery only and 31 with T3 disease who had received adjunctive radiation and found no difference. A small series from New York University also found no difference in local failure whether or not postoperative radiation was given.

For most of these studies, the duration of follow-up is short, yet even in the case of stage T3 tumors, the time to failure after radical prostatectomy may be long.

2. Adjunctive Therapy Directed by Prostate-Specific Antigen

a) After radical prostatectomy, detectable levels of serum prostate-specific antigen warrant consideration of additional therapy on the premise that prostate cancer must be present and that treatment of subclinical small-volume disease might offer the best opportunity for cure or control. Brawer and Lange found that elevations of *PSA above detectable levels will predict recurrence in 100%* patients, whereas *undetectable PSA levels will be associated with a recurrence rate of less than 10%.* Lightner and Lange also reported that pelvic irradiation administered to 26 patients with detectable postprostatectomy PSA resulted in a fall of the marker to undetectable levels in

Table 3. Local control (N° of recurrences / total patients) with irradiation after radical prostatectomy (1-25 years of follow-up)

	TIME OF RADIATION RELATIVE TO RECURRENCE	
	Before (Adjunctive)	After (Therapeutic)
Ray et al[83]	10/13	11/19
Rosen et al[85]	15/16	10/13
Forman et al[20]	12/12	6/6
Hanks and Dawson[36]*	10/10	8/10
Carter et al[12]	30/31	
Gibbons et al[27]*	21/22	
Pilepich et al[80]	18/18	
Lange et al[57]	34/35	
Bahnson et al[3]	14/14	
Fried and Mandell[23]	6/6	
Total	170/177 (96%)	35/48 (73%)

*Hormone therapy used in some patients.

10 cases (38 %). These findings suggest that *marker-producing tissue, PSA production, or both can be eliminated by irradiation.*

b) After irradiation therapy, the source of PSA, unlike the situation with radical prostatectomy, may also be residual resistant tumor within the prostate capsule, de novo tumor developing at some interval after ablation of the original primary, benign prostatic tissue remnants capable of antigen production, or any combination of these. Thus, recommendations for treatment based on prostate-specific antigen levels after irradiation are unclear.

Prospective trials aimed at determining the benefit of adjunctive therapy for high risk patients are in order.

3. Therapeutic Measures

a) Surgery for Radiation Failure:

The experience with surgical excision after irradiation failure is small. A recent report of the experience from the Mayo Clinic reported bladder neck contracture in 17% and incontinence and lymphoedema in 10%. Positive surgical margins were noted in 50% of specimens. Mador and associates performed radical prostatectomy or cystoprostatectomy in seven patients with local failure. They reported rectal laceration in two patients, one of whom developed a fistula. Only two of the cancers were organ confined.

The experience with "salvage" prostatectomy is limited, but thus far, **complications and histologic upstaging discourage widespread application.**

b) Irradiation for Surgical Failure:

A number of investigators have used external-beam irradiation for the treatment of clinical local failure after radical prostatectomy. Ray and associates reported local control in 58% of patients. However, the rate of survival free of disease was only 20% at 6 years. Various investigators have compared the outcome of prophylactic irradiation delivered in high-risk patients before recurrence, with therapeutic irradiation delivered in the setting of clinical recurrence.

As anticipated, the former group experienced better local control and survival. This outcome could be attributed to more effective treatment in the setting of subclinical disease, but conclusions must be tempered by the knowledge that all patients deemed at risk and receiving irradiation will not necessarily develop local failure and by the fact that time interval calculations from treatment to failure are not uniform. Randomized trials are addressing this issue.

c) Antiandrogen Therapy:

Our patients were treated with hormonal therapy **only at the time of failure** of definitive radiation. Of the 48 patients with local failure treated by hormone therapy, 25 (52%) presented no further local growth or complications. This parallels the experience at the Mayo Clinic, where 11 of 22 patients with local failure demonstrated tumor response without further difficulties after hormone therapy.

IV. LOCAL FAILURE AND DISTANT METASTASES

Important to the issue of local control is the incidence of distant metastases and survival. In our radical prostatectomy series, **metastatic disease was found in 5 of 8 (67%) patients with local failure versus 8 of 47 (17%) with local control**. This relation between local and distant failure also exists in irradiation series. Our irradiation data show that within tumor grade and stage, a *statistically higher incidence of distant metastases is associated with failure of control of the primary lesion*. Of those patients with local failure, 68% developed metastases versus 19% of those with locally controlled cancer.

Simultaneous or subsequent distant failure in the patients with local failure *may be caused by dissemination from persistent local tumor*. However, *an alternative explanation* is that the residual local tumor and the distant failure are independent manifestations of *disease of high biologic potential that has already spread at the time of diagnosis and will resist local therapy*.

V. MORBIDITY AND MORTALITY ASSOCIATED WITH LOCAL FAILURE

While **local tumor control** in the presence of distant disease does not alter survival, it may **impact significantly on the quality of survival,** in addition to suppressing a potential source of continuing metastatic dissemination.

Complications can be classified as morbid or lethal.

Morbid complications include unilateral ureteral obstruction, bladder obstruction or incontinence necessitating treatment by transurethral resection or placement of ure-thral or suprapubic catheter, and hematuria requiring intervention for clot evacuation or fulguration.

Lethal complications included bilateral ureteral obstruction and bowel obstruction.

Patients with stage T_1b or stage T_2a tumors treated by any modality have a **negligible incidence** of local failure and virtually no complications secondary to local failure. Patients with **stage T3 tumors have a high incidence of local failure and attendant morbidity or death** with each of the treatment modalities. The difference of importance occurs with stage T_2b tumors, where both external-beam irradiation and radical prostatectomy are associated with statistically fewer complications than was I-125.

When analyzed by grade, **well-differentiated tumors are rarely associated with post-treatment local morbidity or death** regardless of the type of treatment. Among patients with poorly differentiated tumors, there is not a statistically significant difference in morbidity and mortality rates whether treatment is by external-beam radiation, radical prostatectomy, or I-125.

The possible implications of our study for local control and local complications of the *treatment of low-grade, low-stage tumors* are several. First, these tumors are of *low biologic potential* and are extirpated or controlled by *any of the modalities* used. Second, the tumors are not significant threats for disease progression or death within the life expectancy of the host and therefore will behave similarly *regardless of treatment modality*. Third, *follow-up has not yet been long enough for expression of recurrence*.

Conversely, *stage T3 or poorly differentiated tumors* are biologically active and will often escape local control and cause complications regardless of the type of local treatment.

VI. FUTURE CONSIDERATIONS

The development and institution of standard protocols for pathologic examination of radical prostatectomy specimens will be necessary to provide a common basis for comparative study.

Improved **detection of seminal vesicle involvement** by ultrasound imaging and guided biopsy may identify patients at exceptionally high risk for failure. Evaluation of **tumor ploidy** by flow cytometric study or image analysis also promises to **identify biologically active tumors at the time of diagnosis.**

Ultrasound-guided isotope placement will avoid some of the difficulties of asymmetrical free-hand seed distribution and nonhomogeneous radiation dosing. The use of **mixed-beam neutron therapy** promises a greater certainty of local control.

The identification of **markers** that can reveal an individual tumor to be particularly **resistant or sensitive to a specific form of therapy** poses a significant challenge.

DOCUMENTATION

BAHNSON RR, GARNETT JE, GRAYHACK JT: Adjuvant radiation therapy in stages C and D1 prostatic adenocarcinoma: Preliminary results. Urology 27.403,1986.

COX LD, STOFFEL TL: The significance of needle biopsy after irradiation for stage C adenocarcinoma of the prostate. Cancer 40:156, 1977.

GEE WF, COLE LR: Symptomatic stage C : of prostate: Traditional therapy. Urology 15:335, 1980.

HANKS GE, DAWSON AK: The role of external beam radiation therapy after prostatectomy for prostate cancer. Cancer 58:2406, 1986.

HOLM HH, JUUL N, PEDERSEN LF, et al: Transperineal 125 iodine seed implantation in prostati(cancer guided by transrectal ultrasonography. J. Urol. 130:283, 1983.

KABALIN LN, HODGE KK, MCNEAL JE, et al: Identification of residual cancer in prostate following radiation therapy: Role of transrectal ultrasound guided biopsy and prostate specific antigen. J. Urol. 142:326, 1989.

KLEIN FA, ALI MM, HACKLER RH: Bilateral pelvic lymphadenectomy, transperineal interstitial implantation of iridium-192 and external beam radiotherapy for advanced localized prostatic carcinoma: Toxicity and early results. Oncol 2:23, 1986.

LIPSETT LA, COSGROVE MD, GREEN N, et al: Factors influencing prognosis in the radiotherapeutic management of carcinoma of the prostate. Int. J. Radiat Oncol Biol Phys 1:1049, 1976.

RAY GR, BAGSHAW MA, FREIHA F: External beam radiation salvage for residual or recurrent local tumor following radical prostatectomy. J Urol 132:926, 1984.

SCHELLHAMMER PF, WHITMORE RB, KUBAN DA, et al: Morbidity and mortality of local failure after definitive therapy for prostate cancer. J Urol 141:567, 1989.

WHITMORE WF, ROSENBERG S, CHOPP R: Wait and see: Experience with B1 lesions. In Prostate Cancer, Part B: Imaging Techniques, Radiotherapy, Chemotherapy, and Management Issues. New York, Alan R Liss, 1987.

Significance and Treatment of Positive Margins or Seminal Vesicle Invasion After Radical Prostatectomy

James E. Montie

Department of Urology, Cleveland Clinic Florida, Ft. Lauderdale, Florida, USA

Directing therapy for localized prostate carcinoma is a difficult task. To make sense out of conflicting results for apparently similar patient groups or apparently similar results obtained with a variety of treatments, the problem must be broken down into manageable issues. Selection of representative but specific clinical circumstances allows examination of data available from a specific therapy. This review examines the impact of local extension of prostate cancer on the outcomes of treatment.

CASE 1

An asymptomatic 60-year-old man has a clinical stage T2b prostate cancer.

The serum PSA concentration is 12.8 ng/ml.

Biopsy identifies a cancer of Gleason score 7 in both lobes. A bone scan is normal.

A radical prostatectomy and pelvic lymphadenectomy are performed. No gross extension of the cancer is evident during removal.

Lymph nodes are negative on frozen section.

*The final pathology examination shows **penetration of the cancer through the capsule. The margin does not appear to be involved.***

I. WHAT OUTCOMES ARE IMPORTANT IN THIS CASE?

The most important finding in this case is the extension through the capsule.

The questions of importance are:

- the risk of **local recurrence,**

- the likelihood of **disease-free survival,** and

- the **morbidity from treatment** (stricture, incontinence, impotence).

1. What is the prostate capsule?

The prostate "capsule" is an entity that causes some controversy among pathologists. The structure is really **only a band of fibromuscular stroma** that lies between the glandular units and the periprostatic loose connective tissue. It is **incomplete**, being **absent at the apex and anteriorly**, and really inseparable from the prostate.

Involvement of this outer margin has been categorized into **three layers**:

- **level III** is penetration into **periprostatic tissue** or smooth muscle of bladder neck

- **level II** is an intact capsular surface but **tumor within two or three cell diameters of the surface,**

- **level I** is all **lesser degrees** of capsular involvement (Fig. 1).

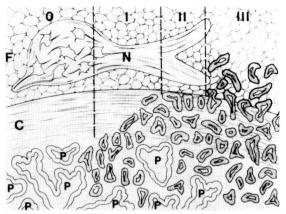

Figure 1. Three levels of capsular involvement of the prostate. (From Stamey et al with permission)

Data indicate that involvement *less than level III probably does not adversely affect local recurrence rates or disease-free survival*, and thus additional local treatment is not necessary.

The Stanford group has recently published a study including 156 clinical stage T2 carcinomas. Capsular penetration was identified in 50% of the cases. In half of these, the *capsular penetration consisted exclusively of perineural space penetration* in nerves immediately external to the capsule. Among the other half of cases, perineural space penetration through the capsule, along with direct penetration through the capsule, was seen in 35. Thus, in only 5% cases was the capsular penetration devoid of perineural space invasion.

This study also examined positive surgical margins based on inked specimens: it appears that the relative absence of a capsule near the apex and the propensity to extend to the margin with perineural space invasion, even with small cancers, makes *the apex the area of highest risk for incomplete removal and positive surgical margins*.

Paulson and associates also made the distinction between extension through the capsule or *specimen-confined* (31%) versus *positive surgical margins* (21%). Clearly, these distinctions must be related to the amount of cancer outside the confines of the prostate, ranging from a few cells identified only in step-sectioning to gross extension seen by the surgeon.

Until a better method becomes available, it would seem that the practice of inking the outside surface of the specimen is helpful. *Tumors extending to the inked surgical margin could be classified as margin positive.*

The urologist is wise to review this issue specifically with the pathologist to be sure there is no confusion in semantics.

2. How often are capsular penetration and positive margins found?

Catalona and Dresner found that 12 of 25 *(48%)* patients with clinical stage *T2b* disease had positive margins defined by established periprostatic soft-tissue involvement (negative lymph nodes). *Data on both extremes of this observation are available*. Middleton and Smith found *only a 12%* incidence of "capsular invasion" (? capsular penetration) in clinical T2b (negative lymph node) patients. Eggleston and Walsh found a *68%* incidence of capsular penetration but thought the margins were positive in only seven cases (6%).

3. How to identify capsular penetration preoperatively?

The capsule cannot be identified consistently by transrectal ultrasonography. Scardino and associates have proposed the term *"boundary echo"* to refer to the hypoechoic border around the outside of the prostate. In addition to true disruption that might be caused by a cancer, there are *many sonographic artifacts* that can give the appearance of irregularity or disruption in this pattern.

More importantly, the *pathologic correlations with the transrectal ultrasonogra-*

phy findings are misleading. In his study, the preoperative transrectal ultrasonography identified discontinuity of the boundary echo in 19; however, the radical prostatectomy specimen showed *extracapsular extension at the site of disruption on ultrasound in only 4 (21%)*.

II. IS TREATMENT NECESSARY FOR EXTRAPROSTATIC EXTENSION?

In 1987, Walsh stated: *"Just because the surgical margins are positive does not mean the patient has residual tumor."* It is unlikely that such an optimistic viewpoint as this would be proposed in another area of surgical oncology. *Residual cancer presumably leads to local recurrences*, but the time to identification of these recurrences in prostate cancer may be extremely protracted, and *disease may not become apparent clinically in the patient's lifetime.*

The limitations of reliable data on local recurrence after radical prostatectomy greatly hinder the drawing of conclusions.

1) A defensible figure for the *local recurrence rate* for clinical T2-pathologic T3 cancers is in the range of 10% to 30%. The influence of periprostatic invasion compared with positive surgical margins is debatable.

2) The *impact of local failure* is often difficult to quantitate because local failure may be discovered simultaneously with distant relapse. Did the local failure lead to the distant relapse, or are aggressive cancers, that are likely to metastasize, also likely to persist locally? *Irrespective of further local treatment, these patients would be destined to do poorly.*

3) However, a logical approach is that failure to eliminate the cancer is evidence of a *failure of the original goal of the treat-*

ment. If the surgical technique could be modified or additional treatment given to decrease local failures, this approach should not be disregarded, although additional morbidity must be carefully weighed against benefit.

III. IS TREATMENT EFFECTIVE FOR EXTRAPROSTATIC EXTENSION?

Two variables can be studied: local recurrence rate and disease free survival.

1. Endocrine therapy can be applied in the setting described in this particular case, but interpretable data are few. This specific approach *will need to be tested*, examining the cost and morbidity of androgen suppression versus the benefit to survival, because only a small percentage of patients are destined to relapse.

2. Radiation therapy after radical prostatectomy appears to be associated with a *lower pelvic recurrence rate*. It would appear that the local recurrence rate can be reduced **to *5% or less***. It is conceivable that local recurrences are only being delayed, not eliminated, but there are no specific data to suggest this.

The effect of postoperative radiation therapy in *preventing systemic recurrences is less clear*. Walsh emphasized the logical concept that many of the cancers that have penetrated the capsule have already produced metastases that often will be manifest and fatal before a local recurrence will become problematic.

Additional local treatment in any form will not appreciably alter survival in such cases. The intermediate disease-free survival rate (approximately 5 years) is approximately 70%, but later follow-up **continues to identify relapses**.

III. IS POSTOPERATIVE RADIATION THERAPY SAFE?

Combining two local treatment modalities *can enhance cumulative toxicity*. In early therapeutic protocols, lymphedema of the genitalia or lower extremities was a serious concern.

1. If the patient has a postoperative *complication from the radical prostatectomy*, namely, vesical neck contracture or an element of incontinence, *radiation will only aggravate the problem and may make it much more difficult to treat*. Most vesical neck contractures are easily dilated or incised without long-term morbidity, but subjection of this stricture to radiation can make it very difficult to manage. In addition, moderate stress incontinence can become appreciably worse, and correction with an artificial sphincter may be difflcult, after irradiation.

Thus, the lesson to be learned is to delay the radiation therapy until the postoperative recovery is complete, usually 2 to 4 months.

2. Doses of radiation in excess of 6500 to 7000 cGy are probably associated with higher complication rates; in addition, because only microscopic disease is being treated, such doses probably are not necessary.

CASE 2

A similar patient is likewise found to have involvement of the seminal vesicles on pathology review. All gross tumor was removed, but the seminal vesicles were noted to be indurated during the operation.

Seminal vesicle invasion has classically been linked to an **incurable situation.** In 1972, Jewett stated "apparently local extension of the tumor into the connective tissue around the seminal vesicles makes surgical cure unlikely". The classic Johns Hopkins philosophy was that seminal vesicle invasion was distinctly worse than capsular penetration alone.

More recent data support the association of seminal vesicle invasion with a higher incidence of positive nodes, earlier systemic relapse, and a greater risk of local recurrence.

Wheeler at Baylor has proposed a *classification system for seminal vesicle invasion* based on the pattern of extension (Fig. 2) seen in 30 cases found among 122 radical prostatectomies:

• **Type I** invasion, defined as extension along the *ejaculatory complex*, was seen in **40%** .

• **Type IIa**, *direct extension* between the base of the prostate and seminal vesicle, was seen in **13%** .

• **Type IIb**, extension **along nerves** in the periprostatic and periseminal vesicle soft tissue and then into the seminal vesicle, was seen in **17%.**

Type II is probably the type most frequently identified in the older literature from which most conclusions relative to survival have been drawn.

- **Type III**, *isolated foci* in the seminal vesicles without involvement of the ejaculatory complex or the presence of adjacent extracapsular tumor, was seen in **30%**.

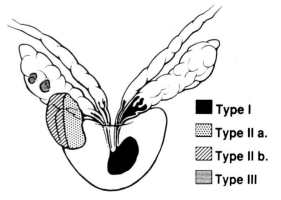

■ Type I
▨ Type II a.
▧ Type II b.
▤ Type III

Figure 2. Three types of seminal vesical invasion; (from Wheeler et al with permission)

In most cases (78%), the section of seminal vesicle near the prostate demonstrated the involvement.

In many centers, the approach to larger cancers of the clinical T2-3 stage is *aggressive surgical therapy*: periprostatic soft-tissue involvement or positive margins are observed and it may be apparent in the operating room that the cancer is invading the bladder neck and extending into the soft tissue and that *cancer is being left behind.* In this circumstance, there is less debate about the potential for local, symptomatic recurrences, and *a stronger case can be made for postoperative radiation* to lessen this risk. On the other hand, these cancers are also more aggressive in general, likely to be associated with nodal metastases and later distant disease, and it is *less probable that better local control will have a salutary effect on survival.*

VI. PERSPECTIVE

◆ **1)** The periprostatic soft-tissue involvement described in the traditional urologic literature is different from that recognized now in 50% of the radical prostatectomy cases. *A much "earlier" pathologic stage T3 is being identified:* a concomitant *improvement in survival* may be seen that will be *only a reflection of "stage migration."*

◆ **2)** In spite of the tiny margin of soft tissue that is able to be removed in a typical radical prostatectomy, *apparent microscopic extension of the cancer to the margin* of the specimen yields a modestly *low risk for a local recurrence*, approximately 25 %.

◆ **3)** *Postoperative radiation is apparently effective in decreasing local recurrences.* If patients are selected properly by avoiding treatment in those with a surgical complication (stricture or incontinence), the treatment is well tolerated. A salutary effect of postoperative adjuvant radiation on *overall survival has not yet been identified.*

◆ **4)** New observations in the *pathologic examination of the specimen* need to be refined. Several questions need to be answered:

a) Is *tumor in the apical area* particularly likely to penetrate into the periprostatic fat, thus yielding a positive surgical margin?

b) Is most periprostatic penetration associated with *perineural space invasion*?

c) Are specific *types of seminal vesicle* involvement *distinguishable*, and if so, what is their significance?

Until the results of the **Intergroup Study on Postoperative Radiation Therapy** are available to give better guidance, *such radiation may best be restricted to patients who have a substantial amount of cancer in the periprostatic soft tissue or involvement of the seminal vesicles, bladder neck, or apical margin.*

DOCUMENTATION

ANSCHER MS, PROSNITZ LR: Postoperative radiotherapy for patients with carcinoma of the prostate undergoing radical prostatectomy with positive surgical margins, seminal vesicle involvement and/or penetration through the capsule. J Urol 138:1407,1987.

GIBBONS RP, COLE BS, RICHARDSON EG, et al: Adjuvant radiotherapy following radical prostatectomy: Results and complications. J Urol 135:65, 1986.

JACOBSON GM, SMITH JA JR, STEWART JR: Postoperative radiation therapy for pathologic stage C prostate cancer. Int J Radiat Oncol Biol Phys 13:1021,1987.

LANGE PH, MOON TD, NARAYAN P: Radiation therapy as adjuvant treatment after radical prostatectomy: Patient tolerance and preliminary results. J Urol 136:45, 1986.

MUKAMEL E, DEKERNION JB, HANNAH J, et al: The incidence and significance of seminal vesicle invasion in patients with adenocarcinoma of the prostate. Cancer 59 : 1335, 1987.

SCARDINO PT, SKIVOHARA K, WHEELER TM, et al: Staging of prostate cancer: Value of ultrasonography. Urol Clin North Am 16:713, 1989.

The role of salvage prostatectomy after radiotherapy failure

P. Link and F.S Freiha

Urology, 37, 189 (1991)

Radiotherapy is credited in the treatment of localized carcinoma of the prostate by its promotors of overall survival rates close to the expected survival rates in the age-matched control population.

However there is a significant rate of local failures which may not be as benign as was once thought. In such cases, therapeutic options are: interstitial irradiation, hormone manipulation or salvage radical prostatectomy.

In order to assess the feasibility, and the rate of complications of salvage prostatectomy, we reviewed the Stanford experience with this procedure.

I- MATERIALS AND METHODS

Of 250 total radical prostatectomies done at Stanford University Medical Center, 14 were performed as a salvage procedure after local failure of external beam radiation therapy (10 patients) or interstitial irradiation (4 patients). The failure had been detected an average of 5 years after the completion of radiation therapy.

II- RESULTS

1- Technicals aspects

a) Preoperative preparation: we routinely prescribed a full bowel preparation, peri-operative antibiotics and anti-embolic stockings.

b) Surgical problems:

- in 10 of 14 cases we encountered a dense fibrosis, making operative dissection more difficult, blunting planes around the prostate, especially between this organ and the rectum. However, their was no rectal injury.

- in all cases, both neurovascular bundles were deliberately excised widely.

- there was no significant difference between salvage and first line radical prostatectomies performed in this department over the same period, regarding blood loss (1000 cc versus 1100 cc) or operating time (185 min versus 175 min).

2. Postoperative course:

a) **final pathology** of the radical salvage prostatectomy specimens showed an average cancer volume of 11.1 cc, capsular penetration in 9 patients (64%), seminal vesicles involvement in 7 patients (50%) and positive margins in 6 patients (43%)

b) immediate course was indistinguishable from that of the first line prostatectomies in terms of early complications, duration of urethral catheterization or hospital stay.

c) long term complications included erectile dysfunction in all patients, which is consistent with the sacrifice of both neurovascular bundles. Post radiation therapy preoperative continence was very satisfactory. Yet, a significant incontinence developped in 6 of the 11 patients (54%) followed for a long enough period of time, as opposed to only 4% in the overall radical prostatectomy series.

d) cancer control: 3 patients received adjuvant external beam radiation therapy and 2 patients had an orchiectomy: 6 patients are free of disease with an average follow-up of 9 months. These 6 patients include 5 of the 7 patients whose seminal vesicles were not involved and one pT3 patient. 4 patients have an elevated PSA without evidence of distance metastasis, with an average follow-up of 14 months.

III- CONCLUSION

From this series of 14 patients we can draw the following conclusions:

1. Salvage radical prostatectomy after local failure of external beam or interstitial irradiation *can be accomplished in a way not much different from first line prostatectomy.*

2. *Post-operative incontinence is significantly more frequent* and erectile dysfunction is constant after post irradiation prostatectomy.

3. *Seminal vesicles involvement* on the salvage prostatectomy specimen is associated with a *high failure rate* of the salvage surgery. We obtain at the present time a very thorough preoperative transrectal ultrasound assessment, so as to offer salvage surgery only if the seminal vesicles appear not to be involved.

4. Our *general impression,* after reviewing this series of 14 patients, is that *there is a role for salvage radical prostatectomy* after local failure of radiation therapy, in patients who are *good surgical risks*, in whom distant *metatasis* and s*eminal vesicles involvement* have been *ruled out.*

5. Nevertheless, the benefit gained in terms of *cancer control cannot be assessed* from this series with a relatively short follow up. It will only be determined by *long term comparative studies.*

IV

STAGE T3 (C)

Management of Stage C (T3-T4) Adenocarcinoma of the Prostate

John H. Lynch, M.D.
Division of Urology, Georgetown University, USA

Prostate cancer is discovered in over 120,000 men in the U.S. each year. Of these, 9% to 15% will have clinical stage C disease at initial staging, and their disease carries a 50% five year mortality. There is a recent trend toward earlier detection, and survival for locally extensive disease may be improving. However, there is no single treatment plan which has risen above the others as the definitive way to treat stage C prostate cancer.

I. NATURAL HISTORY

The natural history of prostate cancer has been studied by observing the progression of untreated patients and by interpreting pathological data from prostatectomy and necropsy specimens.

A Swedish study in which localized prostate cancer (T1-2) patients were observed until progression without therapy showed a 72% five-year disease free survival and a 94% 5 year disease specific survival. The rate of progression to T3 or metastatic disease was much higher in patients with poorly-differentiated cancers than in patients with well-differentiated lesions. The authors urge that the low rate of progression, especially with well-differentiated cancers, become the baseline against which studies of therapy be compared.

Pathologic studies of prostate cancer specimens has led to speculation on the behavior of cancers. There is a direct correlation between cancer volume, local extension and metastatic disease; any one of these factors carries a 50% 8-year progression rate. High grade is correlated with all of the poor prognostic indicators and with progression. Essentially all cancers over 12 cc. in volume have all of the other poor prognostic features present. On the other hand, tumors less than 4 cc. rarely metastasize.

The **extent of capsular involvement** by cancer has prognostic significance, with minimal involvement having little effect on survival, and capsular perforation equalling seminal vesicle involvement as a prognostic indicator. There is one report that less than 1 cm length of capsular perforation may not adversely effect survival. Using the nerve-sparing technique, Stamey et al. found that one half of capsular penetrations were at the prostatic apex, one-fourth on the posterior or lateral sides, and one-fourth at the bladder neck or superior pedicle. Almost all of the apical extensions were along the nerve bundles in the inferior pedicles.

The likelihood of a tumor invading the **seminal vesicles** is related to its proximity to the prostatic midbase; the route of invasion is along the muscular wall of the ejaculatory duct rather than through the capsule.

II. STAGING

Most recent data on staging errors are derived from pathological correlations of patients with clinically localized disease who undergo radical prostatectomies with lymph node dissections.

Understaging of patients is frequent: local extension is found rarely in stage AI, 11% to 50% of clinical stage A2 patients, 17% to 33% of B1 patients, and 39% to 66% of B2 patients. In pathological T3 patients (pT3), positive lymph nodes were found in about 50% of patients; they were found more commonly when seminal vesicle invasion was present than when capsular perforation alone was present. In comparison, positive lymph nodes were discovered in 39% to 56% of patients with clinical stage C disease. Pathological downstaging of stage C patients has been reported to be as high as 30%.

The accepted workup of patients discovered to have carcinoma of the prostate is a digital rectal examination, tissue diagnosis usually by needle biopsy of the prostate (except Stage A), serum prostate specific antigen and prostatic acid phosphatase levels, a chest X-ray and a bone scan. Many practitioners incorporate transrectal sonogram, CT and/or MRI into their evaluation. Diagnostic lymph node dissections are performed routinely with radical retropubic. prostatectomy or independently before non-operative therapy. Despite all these measures, staging errors occur too frequently.

1. Digital Rectal Examination (DRE)

Digital rectal examination (DRE) is the most prevalent prostate examination in use because it is cheap, easily performed and readily available to any practitioner with a knowledgeable finger. Induration extending into either or both lateral sulci or induration into the seminal vesicles is evidence of local extension. The majority of stage B and some stage C cancers are discovered by DRE. Unfortunately, the finger discriminates poorly between stage B and early stage C lesions, and it cannot predict accurately the size of tumor nodules.

2. Transrectal Ultrasound of the Prostate (TRUS)

Transrectal ultrasound of the prostate (TRUS) has been most useful in the diagnosis of prostate cancer where it is helpful in evaluating patients with abnormal prostates by DRE and patients with an elevated PSA level, and in directing needle biopsies. At present, it is not generally being used in the routine screening of adult men.

Studies evaluating TRUS as a staging tool vary in their conclusions. Palken et al. found TRUS unable to measure tumor volume to within 25% in most patients, and it failed to identify local extension in 10 of 11 patients. Others evaluating TRUS for local extension have reported sensitivities of 57% to 86% with specificities of 71% to 100%.

These two studies report a specificity of 100%, suggesting that when local invasion is seen, it reliably diagnoses stage C disease. TRUS can direct systematic biopsies of the prostate and seminal vesicles to improve staging accuracy.

Several **TRUS characteristics of capsular penetration** have been described:

• tumor volume greater than 3 cc;

• loss of normal contour of the capsule;

and obliteration of the trapezoid bounded by the prostatic apex, the urethra, the rectal wall and the rectourethralis muscle.

Seminal vesicle changes are more subtle and include focal alterations in the echogenicity, anterior displacement, asymmetry, and loss of the "beak" where the seminal vesicle joins the ejaculatory duct.

3. Computerized Tomography (CT) and Magnetic Resonance Imaging (MRI).

CT scanning has performed poorly in the evaluation of local extension and **lymph node metastases** in prostate cancer patients. Overall accuracy in assessing local extension is 58% to 65% and in assessing lymph node metastases is 0% to 75%. In one study, only one patient in 21 had improved staging over DRE by CT and MRI.

Determination of local extension by **MRI** is 64% to 86% accurate, which is marginally better than results by CT scanning. Identification of lymph nodes is poor because of the high incidence of microscopic metastases to pelvic lymph nodes.

4. Prostate Specific Antigen (PSA)

Most of the data published about PSA shows that it is nominally useful in staging prostate cancer patients. Each gram of cancer contributes approximately 3.5 ng/ml to the PSA level, while a gram of benign prostate adenoma raises PSA 0.3 ng/ml. **PSA levels are highly correlated with extent of disease**, capsular penetration, seminal vesicle invasion, and metastases. However, cutoff levels for locally invasive or metastatic disease could not be found that differentiated between these stages accurately. Others found that a **PSA less than 10 ng/ml** was highly predictive of negative lymph nodes on examination, whereas a **PSA greater than 50 ng/ml** corresponded to a 90% to 100% seminal vesicle involvement rate and a 20% to 66% lymph node involvement rate. While PSA levels are suggestive of cancer volume and stage, categorical levels for separating tumor stages do not exist.

Metastatic cancer rarely exists with a PSA < 10 ng/ml. A Mayo Clinic study found less than 1% of patients with PSA less than 20 ng/ml had positive bone scans. They and others recommend against getting routine bone scans in patients with PSA less than 10 ng/ml.

5. Prostatic Acid Phosphatase (PAP)

PAP has gained acceptance as a sensitive indicator of metastatic disease on initial evaluation. 66% of D1 and 94% of D2 patients have elevated PAP. It is elevated in 34% to 64% of patients with clinical stage C disease. Whitesel et al. introduced the term "D0" in 1984, stating that an elevated PAP heralded metastatic disease even if no metastasis could be clinically demonstrated. 60% of these had positive nodes at operation, and 88% of patients followed 2 years developed metastatic disease. This study was criticized because the treatment of patients was not standardized, but the "D0" term and significance have endured.

Recent studies by Stamey have refuted the predictive value of PAP for metastatic disease. 22% of stage A and B patients had elevated PAP. PSA was significantly more sensitive to tumor volume, local tumor extension and metastatic disease than was PAP.[7]

6. DNA Ploidy

The predictive value of DNA ploidy for recurrence is stronger than the presence of seminal vesicle invasion in one study. The five-year disease free survival rate was 85% for diploid tumors and 9% for aneuploid tumors. The predictive power of ploidy was sustained after the effects of seminal vesicle invasion and Gleason's score were eliminated.

7. Lymphangiogram

In studies comparing lymphangiogram to lymph node dissection, lymphangiogram had a false positive rate of 60% and a false negative rate of 20% to 36%. Today it is rarely employed in the evaluation of prostate cancer.

8. Lymph Node Dissection

A pathological specimen is undoubtedly the most accurate way for assessing the status of lymph nodes. Using a modified sampling technique with intra-operative frozen sectioning, the Johns Hopkins group found a 12% node positive rate of which only 2% were grossly positive. Frozen sectioning discovered 67% of the microscopic-only nodes. When the dissection is limited to the space between the external and internal iliac veins, and subsequent radical prostatectomy or radiation therapy is used, a major complication rate of about 7% is reported, including pulmonary emboli, deep venous thrombosis and nerve palsies. Minor complications occurred in an additional 15%.

There are several recent advances in the technique of lymph node dissection. A preliminary report of examining PSA levels in homogenized lymph nodes intra-operatively may decrease the delay and improve the sensitivity over standard techniques of frozen sectioning. Laparoscopic lymph node dissections is being used primarily in academic centers.

In stage C cancer, where 46% are likely to have occult positive nodes, some authors have used lymph node dissections for staging prior to initiating radiation or surgical therapy. The accuracy of a pathological diagnosis is unsurpassed by any other modality; the morbidity of inappropriate treatment in the patient with undiscovered metastatic disease must be weighed against that of the lymph node dissection.

9. Bone Scan

Nuclear medicine bone scanning is the accepted modality for assessing metastatic disease beyond the level of pelvic lymph nodes, and it is routinely employed in the initial evaluation of prostate cancer patients and for follow-up evaluations of disease progression. Bone scan replaced bone surveys early in the last decade when it was determined to be the cheaper, safer and more sensitive procedure. Only 7% of patients with an elevated PAP had negative bone scans versus 22% for bone surveys.

Recent reports show that **PSA levels of less than 10** are never associated with positive bone scans, and that **PSA levels less than 20** are associated with negative bone scans in 99% of patients. These authors suggest that the use of bone scan should be curtailed in these patients. In addition, in post-treatment patients, *a rise in PSA was always seen before metastatic progression could be found by bone scan*.

III. TREATMENT

The current therapy rendered to patients with clinical or pathological stage C prostate cancer runs the gamut of options available to all stages of the disease. Deciphering which treatment option is the best for all or for a particular patient is frought with difficulty because of the inaccuracies in clinical staging and the inability to find matched series with which to compare results. In addition are the facts that stage C is associated with only a 50% five year survival, and the majority of patients are eventually treated with hormonal therapy, thus confusing survival statistics. Examination of the American College of Surgeons Patterns of Care Study reveals a shift in the 80's toward more radiotherapy and away from hormonal therapy and away from a combination of surgery and hormonal therapy in patients with clinical stage C prostate cancer. As we evolve in the 90's the pendulum seems to be swaying back toward combination therapy, including earlier hormonal therapy, and away from radiotherapy by itself.

1. Radiation

a) External beam

The rationale supporting the use of external beam radiotherapy for disease extending beyond the confines of the capsule is the fact that the *fields can be changed to include local diseased areas*. Thus, radiotherapy has the potential to treat what would be considered to be *beyond the margins of the surgical cure*.

Again, *assessment of the results of radiotherapy* are a problem because of the inaccuracy of clinical staging of local disease as well as the uncertainty of nodal involvement in the radiotherapy series.

The treatment of 551 patients with clinical stage C prostate cancer at M. D. Anderson between 1965 and 1982 has been reported. These patients had varying degrees of disease beyond the prostate (Cl and C2) but no evidence of lymphatic or hematogenous metastases. Overall survival rates were 72%, 47% and 27% at 5, 10 and 15 years. Local control rates were 88%, 81% and 75% of 5, 10 and 15 years. They also showed no statistical difference in local control based on dosages. Treatment techniques varied over the years as a matter of policy and most all patients were eventually treated with endocrine manipulation. Stanford reports 61%, 36% and 22%, 5-, 10-, and 15-year survivals respectively (Table 1).

The *issue of local control* is an important, although complicated one. In those patients who exhibit a positive biopsy following radiotherapy, disease progression tends to occur sooner and more frequently. Schellhammer et al. found a post-radiation positive biopsy rate of 39%. Kiesling reported a 58% positive rate while the Mayo Clinic study of 39 patients had a local failure rate of 41%. While the incidence of "local failure" might seem high, Gibbons et al. reports only 8% of 209 patients required subsequent surgery for release of obstruc-

tion. Criteria for "local control" vary among series, and one must be careful whether this refers to biopsy only or clinical evidence of local disease producing symptoms.

External beam radiotherapy is tolerated fairly well. The incidence of *moderate complications* ranges from 9% to 23%, while the incidence of *severe complications* is approximately 6.7%. In the M.D. Anderson study, 23% of patients had anorectal symptoms, and 17% had urinary symptoms.

2. Interstitial radiotherapy

In 1985, Memorial Sloan Kettering Cancer Center reported the results in treating patients with interstitial Iodine. There were 143 patients with clinical stage C cancer; during follow-up periods ranging from 2 to 10 years, 18% had local recurrence only, while 55% had distant metastases (with or without local disease). The 5 year survival rate was 59%. There was a distinct difference in recurrence rate between high grade and low grade lesions (98% high grade) and a distinct survival difference between Cl and C2 disease (69%, 13%). Schellhammer reported a 4% local failure rate for stage C prostate cancer patients treated with interstitial Iodine 125, higher than the 28% reported following external beam (Table 2).

The Baylor group, using a combination of Au-I98 interstitial therapy and external beam radiotherapy, reported a 51% disease-free survival at 5 years and 23% at 10 years for clinical stage C patients. This treatment was not used in clinical stage C2 patients, thus making comparison difficult.

One of the perceived problems with interstitial radiotherapy has been the difficulty of *accurate seed placement* to assure the delivery of an adequate dosage to the tumor burden. With improvement in ultrasound tech-

Table 1. External beam radiotherapy for clinical stage C

Name	5 Yr	10 Yr	15 Yr	Local control
Mason Clinic	57%	31%		
Mayo	77%			86%
Stanford	61%	36%	22%	
M.D. Anderson	72%	47%	27%	75%
Mallinrodt	65%	35%		60%

Table 2. Interstitial radiotherapy for clinical stage C

Name	5 Yr	10 Yr	15 Yr	Local control
MSKCC	59%			18% (I-125)
Schellhammer				44% (I-125)
Baylor	51%	23%		62% (Au-198)
Loening				50% (perineal)

niques, there seems to be an increasing interest in resurrecting interstitial radiation treatment using the *perineal approach with ultrasound guidance*. There are no long term studies to assess survival, but local control continues to be a problem with 50% positive post-treatment biopsy results reported.

The use of interstitial radiotherapy in clinical stage C as sole treatment does not seem to offer any advantages over external beam radiotherapy but may benefit selected patients as combination therapy.

3. Transurethral Resection

Transurethral prostatectomy has certainly been employed in patients with clinical stage C prostate cancer, usually for relief of symptoms caused by outlet obstruction instead of for primary therapy of the malignancy. Hanks reported a significant negative impact on survival on stage C patients who are initially diagnosed by TURP rather than by needle biopsy. His series, however, does not take into account volume of disease or presence of symptoms. For example, are most patients who undergo TURP really stage C2 since they have si-

gnificant outflow obstruction? The Mayo Clinic reported that while TURP is associated with a decrease in local control, TURP has no impact on prognosis, regardless of the grade. Paulson reported on 145 patients undergoing radical prostatectomy to address the issue of tumor spread by TURP. Cancer dianosis was established by TURP in 33 and by needle biopsy in 100. No increase in metastatic disease could be identified in the group who underwent TURP prior to prostatectomy. *Thus, the potential negative impact of TURP on survival has not been proven.*

4. Radical Surgery

As with other modalities, it is difficult to interpret results of surgical series dealing with stage C disease because of the inclusion of other treatment modalities as adjuvant therapy. Zincke et al. reported on 101 patients with clinical stage C lesions undergoing radical prostatectomy. Patients with subtrigonal involvement were excluded. 49 of 101 patients had pathologic stage C tumors while the remainder had 1 or more positive pelvic lymph nodes. Local recurrence occurred in 28% who had no adjuvant treatment but in no patients who had orchiectomy. Orchiectomy, however, had no effect on survival. The observed survival at 5 and 10 years were similar to age-matched controls. Survival rates will be improved or altered significantly only if the surgery can remove all tumor. Bosch reported only 14 of 48 (29%) patients with complete tumor removal defined as negative lymph nodes and negative margins of resection.

Local control rates with radical prostatectomy varied from 8.7% reported by Tomlinson to the 28% reported by Zincke in those patients not receiving adjuvant therapy.

Several reports have addressed the issue of *more extensive surgical procedures* for clinical stage C disease. Spaulding and

Whitmore reported on 37 patients managed by pelvic exenteration or cystoprostatectomy. Local control for stage C lesions was 48%. Of the 35 patients who survived the surgery, 24 died of prostate cancer with only 7 surviving 9 to 20 years with no further evidence of disease. Two patients died following surgery and 18 experienced complications. Many of these patients had previous therapy prior to surgery. Moul and Paulson reported on 22 patients who underwent salvage surgery. 10 of the 22 had no prior therapy. 9 of these 10 were alive at 59 months. Three of the 10 had negative surgical margins. The other 12 patients in the series had surgery for radio-recurrent disease.

9. Hormonal Therapy

The VACURG studies are the only significant studies dealing with hormonal therapy alone in stage C patients. Although there was certainly a delay in progressions to stage D2 (15% and 25% at 5 and 10 years versus 40% and 60% with placebo), there does not appear to be a survival advantage.

There does seem to be **growing interest in the use of hormonal therapy to treat clinical stage C patients** for a variety of reasons.

• A significant percentage of these patients have positive pelvic lymph nodes; therefore, surgical cure may be unlikely.

• Recent radiotherapy data show that a high percentage of patients exhibit positive biopsies and rising PSA's within two years after completion of therapy.

• The NCI study on complete androgen blockade suggests earlier hormonal therapy may prolong survival. In terms of local control, Catalona reported that 68% of patients treated with hormonal therapy had resolution of obstructive symptoms without requiring further local control.

10. Combination Therapy

a) The enthusiasm for **post-radiation radical prostatectomy** or cystoprostatectomy for radio-recurrent disease is reducing as the role of prostatectomy appears to be expanding. Zincke reported on 62 patients with an overall survival of 65% at 5 years and 41% at 10 years. He concluded that radical prostatectomy may have a role following radiation failure in small volume disease but that the wisdom of exenterative procedures for large volume disease seems questionable. In Paulson's series of 12 patients, disease in 41.7% was confined to the surgical specimen. Goldstone and Scardino also had 41% of their series of 28 with negative surgical margins and no seminal vesicle invasion. Rectal injuries occurred in 18%, anastomotic strictures in 21% and complete urinary continence was achieved in only 60%. Thus, although it may be possible to surgically excise all tumor and radio-recurrent disease, the complications are certainly higher, and one must be selective in their indications for such procedures. Gill et al. reported on a "sandwich radiotherapy" in which 15 patients with clinical stage C were treated with 3,000 rads, had prostatectomy, and then received an additional 2,000 rads to the pelvis plus 2,500 rads to the prostatic fossa plus 4,500 rads to the periaortic-cava lymph node area. They have no demonstrable recurrence in the pelvis, but follow-up is only 6 months to 5 1/2 years.

b) Perhaps the most commonly employed combination of therapy today is that of **radical prostatectomy followed by external beam radiotherapy**. It must be remembered that these are typically patients thought to have organ-confined disease but who, on pathologic examination, are found to have positive surgical margins, seminal vesicle involvement or organ-positive but surgical margin negative disease. Post-prostatectomy radiotherapy can reduce PSA levels in

82% of patients and can reduce local recurrences normally in the 25% range to the 0 to 5% range, but there is no confirmed data suggesting a survival advantage.

The other combination generating widespread interest is **preoperative hormonal treatment** in an effort to "down-stage" B2/C disease. Scott and Void reported on this concept in 1969. In their series of 39 selected patients, the overall 5 year survival rate was 74.4% with 61.5% being disease-free. Thirty-three patients were followed for 10 years with a 51% disease free survival. The RTOG conducted a randomized trial from 1983 to 1986, randomizing patients between either Megestrol or DES followed by radiotherapy. Their study showed no advantage for either drug.

Soloway is currently studying a group of 20 patients treated with several months of preoperative hormonal therapy with LHRH agents and Flutamide. Three of twenty had positive nodes, and nine of twenty had margin-positive disease. Six patients have had continuation of androgen deprivation. Although a 30% to 50% size reduction can occur there is no definitive evidence of conversion to organ confined disease.

Thomas, Lowe, Carroll and Narayan recently reported on a group of 24 patients with histologic or imaging evidence of extracapsular or seminal vesical disease. Eighteen were treated with a combination of LHRH analogues and Flutamide, 4 with LHRH analogues alone and 2 with DES. All patients were treated with 3 months of therapy. Although 70% were clinically "downstaged", 35 % had positive nodes confirmed at time of node dissection and 80% had extracapsular disease at the time of surgery. Of the three patients with organ-confined disease, two had pre-op "suggestions" of S.V. invasion and one has a rising PSA. To date, therefore, there is no scientific data to support the use of pre-op hormonal therapy to pathologically down-stage patients with locally advanced disease.

In summary, review of the many series dealing with the treatment of patients with clinical stage C prostate cancer fails to find a single modality or combination or modality superior to any other. Accurate staging was difficult in older studies; stage migration complicates the comparison of recent to older studies. **The majority of patients ultimately progress and are therefore treated with hormonal therapy**, thus obscuring survival. This points to the need for controlof randomized clinical trials to answer these questions in the future.

DOCUMENTATION

ANDRIOLE GL, KAVOUSSI LR, TORRENCE RJ, LEPOR J CATALONA WJ. Transrectal ultrasonography in the diagnosis and staging of carcinoma of the prostate. J Urol 140: 758, 1988.

BEZZI M, KRESSEL HY, ALLEN KS, SCHIEBLER ML, ALTMAN HG WEIN AJ, POLLACK HM. Prostatic carcinoma: staging with MR imaging at l.5TI. Radiology 169: 339, 1988.

CATALONA WJ, STEIN AJ. Staging errors in clinically localized prostatic cancer. J Urol 127: 452, 1982.

CHYBOWSKI FM, KELLER JJL, BERGSTRALH EJ, OESTERLING JE. Predicting radionuclide bone scan findings in patients with newly diagnosed, untreated prostate cancer: prostate specific antigen is superior to all other clinical parameters. J Urol 145: 313, 1991.

KAYE RI, PAUL-BLANC R, WILBUR HJ, LAMONT BM, FISHER HAG. Value of abdominopelvic CT scanning in treatment planning of prostate cancer. AUA Abstract 77, 1990.

LANGE PH, NARAYAN P. Understaging and undergrading of prostate cancer: argument for postoperative radiation as adjuvant therapy.Urology 21: 113, 1983.

LANGE PH, ERCOLE CJ, LIGHTNER DJ, FRALEY EE, VESSELLA R. The value of serum prostate specific antigen determinations before and after radical prostatectomy. J Urol 141: 873, 1989.

MOUL JW, PAULSON DF. The role of radical surgery in the management of large volume T3 and T4 and radiation persistent cancer. AUA Abstract 122, 1990.

OESTERLING JE, CHAN DW, EPSTEIN JI, KIMBALL AW, BRUZEK DJ, ROCK RC, BRENDLER CB, WALSH PC. Prostate specific antigen in the preoperative and postoperative evaluation of localized prostatic cancer treated with radical prostatectomy. J Urol 139: 766, 1988.

SPIGELMAN SS, MCNEAL JE, FREIHA FS, STAMEY TA. Rectal examination in volume determination of carcinoma of the prostate: clinical and anatomical correlations. J Urol 136: 1228, 1986.

STAMEY TA, VILLERS AA, MCNEAL JE, LINK PC, FREIHA FS. Positive surgical margins at radical prostatectomy: importance of apical dissection. J Urol 143: 1166, 1990.

STAMEY TA, KABALIN JN, MCNEAL JE, JOHNSTONE IM, FREIHA F, REDWINE EA, YANG N. Prostate specific antigen in the diagnosis and treatment of adenocarcinoma of the II. Radical prostatectomy treated patients. J Urol 141: 1076, 1989.

WHITESEL JA, DONOHUE RE, et al. Acid phosphatase: its influence on the management of carcinoma of the prostate. J Urol 131: 70, 1984.

V

STAGE N+ (D1)

Management of Stage N+ (D1) Prostate Cancer

Mark S. Austenfeld

Section of Urology, University of Kansas Medical Center, Kansas City, Kansas, USA

Although the treatment of prostate cancer in all stages is controversial, there is perhaps most disagreement with respect to stage N+ disease. Because few randomized prospective studies have been performed, comparison of outcomes is primarily possible through retrospective data. These comparisons are difficult given the extreme variability of prostate cancer behavior and many applied treatment options. A critical review of the published literature to date on stage N+ prostate cancer will be presented here.

I. CLINICAL DATA

1. Demographics

One third of patients at diagnosis have *metastatic disease*.

Of the patients diagnosed with *no evidence of metastasis*, 27% have pelvic lymph node involvement when surgically staged.

2. Staging and diagnosis

Stage N+ prostate cancer most commonly is diagnosed histologically after pelvic lymph node dissection (PLND). Although the overall incidence of pelvic lymph node metastases is about 30% in clinically localized disease, this *rate depends* largely upon the *grade* and *stage* of the primary tumor. High grade clinical stage T3 prostate cancer carries a risk of pelvic nodal involvement of over 90% whereas less than 5% of well-differentiated small clinical stage T2 tumors will have positive nodes.

The majority of patients with *any elevation of enzymatic prostatic acid phosphatase or a serum prostate specific antigen level* greater than 20 nanograms per milliliter will have positive pelvic lymph nodes or seminal vesicle involvement at staging operation. *Size of the primary tumor* and perhaps tumor *DNA aneuploidy* are additionally associated with risk of occult pelvic metastases.

3. Natural history and prognosis

Since the advent of routine node dissection, multiple studies have verified the presence of pelvic lymphatic involvement as an *independent, poor prognostic variable.*

Because most patients receive some form of hormonal deprivation prior to prostate cancer death, data regarding the natural history of stage N+ disease without delayed endocrine treatment are nonexistent.

Therefore, the best means available to evaluate the natural history of stage N+ prostate cancer is through studies that include a cohort of patients with clinically localized cancer found to have positive pelvic lymph nodes after staging node dissection and receiving no initial treatment to the primary tumor. It is observed from studies of these

Table 1. Incidence of positive nodes according to stage.

Tumor	N°	Pos.	%
A1 (T1a)	64	0	0
A2 (T1b)	549	126	23
B1 (T2a)	1,096	144	13
B2 (T2b)	984	275	23
B3 (T2c)	419	94	22
C (T3-T4)	1,380	594	43
TOTALS	**4,492**	**1,233**	**27**

patients that *if left untreated, 75% will progress systemically and 50% will die within five years of their diagnosis.*

4. Influence of positive seminal vesicules, tumor grade, elevated acid phosphatase, volume of nodal disease and ploidy.

Poor tumor differentiation, preoperative elevation of enzymatic prostatic acid phosphatase and the presence of tumor within the seminal vesicles all signal the much greater likelihood that prostate cancer has become a systemic disease. Certainly, the majority of these patients will have nodal involvement upon surgical staging. However, *once the pelvic lymph nodes are involved, these adverse prognostic variables alter the prognosis only slightly* particularly when early hormonal deprivation is instituted.

The prognostic significance of the *volume of tumor within pelvic lymph nodes* is controversial. It is well-documented that when minimal lymph nodes are involved (only one node positive or less than 3 cc total volume), the majority of patients will be alive at five years regardless of treatment. Unfortunately, with extended follow-up these patients frequently progress and their survival after ten years differs little from patients with greater nodal volume.

Recent data from the Mayo Clinic have revealed encouraging evidence that the prognosis of stage N+ cancer patients is accurately predicted through flow cytometric analysis.

II. TREATMENT MONOTHERAPY

1. Surgery

Without adjuvant systemic therapy, surgery to remove the prostate and involved pelvic lymph nodes *does little to prolong survival*. Less than one half of these patients survive progression-free at five years.

Patients with minimal amounts of nodal metastases from prostate cancer treated by surgery as a single modality have a reasonably good five year progression free survival. However, most will progress and many will die of their disease before ten years follow-up.

2. Radiation therapy

Brachytherapy using I-125 *alone has been shown to be ineffective* in the treatment of stage N+ prostate cancer.

Since the development of the *linear accelerator*, external beam radiation has been widely used to treat prostate cancer. Although other authors have reported their results when applying this modality to the whole pelvis of node positive patients, Bagshaw and coworkers have the largest and best staged series within the radiotherapy literature. Of 146 patients who underwent staging pelvic lymph node dissection, 61 were found to have nodal involvement and were treated with extended field radiotherapy. Of these patients, only 50% and 10% were alive at five and ten years, respectively. These patients *did significantly worse than those with negative nodes,* (Figure 1) and appear very similar to the performance of patients followed by observation and delayed hormonal deprivation alone.

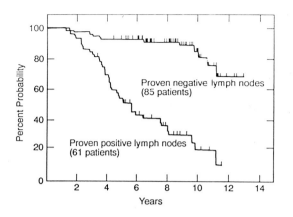

Figure 1. Comparison of survival according to the presence of biopsy-proven lymphatic metastases in patients receiving radiation treatment for prostatic adenocarcinoma. (Bagshaw et al)

3. Early endocrine treatment

The VACURG studies I and II shed some light on the questionable merit of *early versus late* hormonal deprivation in prostate cancer.

Patients with stages C and D (locally advanced and metastatic) were given placebo or various forms of hormonal deprivation. Those treated initially by placebo were often crossed over to hormonal deprivation when significant progression was apparent. Therefore, performance differences between the placebo group and hormonal groups have been more accurately compared as early versus late hormonally treated disease. Although in the original assessment of these data, no survival advantages could be attributed to the early use of endocrine suppression, Byar and Green, using a mathematical model, later published evidence that *early endocrine therapy* may have *advantages* over delayed endocrine therapy *in younger patients with higher grade tumors.*

Kramolowski was able to demonstrate *prolonged time to progression and improved cause-specific survival* (CSS) in 30 patients receiving early endocrine treatment alone or as an adjuvant to various primary therapeutic modalities. The mean time to progression was 100 months with a 5 year CSS of 67% compared to 43 months and 53%, respectively, for the 38 patients receiving delayed endocrine treatment.

4. Chemotherapy

To date, chemotherapy used to treat adenocarcinoma of the prostate has been ineffective. However, *no data exist which adequately assess the effect of chemotherapy alone on stage N+ disease.* Cytotoxic medical therapy may hold some promise when used adjuvantly to treat early systemic disease. Laboratory support of this concept is found in well conducted studies demonstrating the sensitivity to chemotherapy of a metastatic prostate cancer variant of the Dunning rat model. Survival of these rats treated with cyclophosphamide was improved when the drug was begun early in the course of the disease or after surgical debulking.

The role of chemotherapy in treating prostate cancer is still evolving. Although end-stage disease responds poorly to cytotoxic agents, treatment of low volume disease may be a reasonable option in selected patients

5. Multimodality treatment

a) Radiation combined with other treatment

Recently Gervasi and associates reported long-term follow-up on 152 patients diagnosed as having positive pelvic lymph nodes and receiving Au-198 seed implantation. All patients received extended external pelvic irradiation when positive nodes were found. The overall five, ten, and fifteen year survival rates for node positive patients were 65, 32, and 6%, respectively, demonstrating the *marginal benefit of this combination.*

Batata and coworkers reported the ineffective-

Table 2. Outcome of stage D1 prostate cancer

TREATMENT*	No. Patients	Median Interval To Progression Months	3-5 Year Survival %		5-10 Year Survival %	
			Progression-Free	Actual	Progression-Free	Actual
Monotherapy: **						
Delayed Hormonal Deprivation[20,21,22]	71	17	25	52		
Immediate Hormonal Deprivation[40]	30	>45	73	80		
Radical Prostatectomy[13,21,24,30]	170	46	42	82	25	61
External Beam[20,21,22,34,35]	169	20	23	47		19
Interstitial Radiation[29,32,33]	151	12	42	62		14
Combination:						
Radical Prostatectomy, Early Hormonal[13,24,30]	347	NR	84	90	71	78
Radical Prostatectomy, External Beam[28,47]	42	45	62	74		
Radical Prostatectomy, Chemotherapy[46]	12	NR	75	92		

∧   Some figures are based on averages of data in the referenced series.
*   All series include pelvic lymph node dissection prior to treatment.
**   Assumed that all monotherapy patients received hormonal suppression before death.
NR   Not Reached

ness of I-125 when combined with external beam and preoperative hormonal deprivation.

De Vere White and associates in 1983 added early chemotherapy to I-125 for 12 patients with N+ cancer. When comparing these patients to 25 others who did not receive adjuvant chemotherapy, they noted a prolonged time to progression and improved short-term disease-free survival. However, no long-term follow-up was available.

The addition of chemotherapy to definitive external beam radiation was reviewed by Schmidt and coworkers of the National Prostate Cancer Project (NPCP). A recent report revealed improved progression-free survival for patients with N+ prostate cancer treated by external radiation and adjuvant estramustine when compared to a group receiving radiation alone. Long-term benefit, however, has yet to be determined.

b) Radical prostatectomy and adjuvant chemotherapy

Carter and coworkers reported results of treatment on 16 patients with stage N+ disease. All underwent radical prostatectomy and 12 patients additionally received four to eight monthly courses of cyclophosphamide. Radiation was also used to a variable degree in these patients. Hormonal therapy was withheld until evidence of clinical progression. With a mean of 61 months follow up, 82% were alive with no evidence of disease. However, only seven patients had been followed at least five years.

c) Prostatectomy and pelvic radiation

Cure by radiation to the whole pelvis in patients with positive nodes after prostatectomy has been attempted. Long-term follow-up to fully evaluate the influence of adjuvant pelvic radiation is not available. **Complications** associated with radiation to the pelvis after lymph node dissection have been published and **must be carefully weighed against any putative benefit.**

c) Prostatectomy and early adjuvant hormonal therapy

Most clinical data showing benefit to early versus delayed hormonal deprivation as an adjuvant to radical prostatectomy come from the Mayo Clinic. Zincke recently updated the **Mayo Clinic experience** on 380 patients treated since 1967. The 294 patients receiving adjuvant early hormonal treatment had five and ten year progression-free survival of 80 and 77%. These patients fared significantly better than 86 patients receiving radical prostatectomy alone with 41 and 22% five and ten year progression-free survival. Perhaps more importantly, **the cause-specific survival rates are beginning to appear better for the early endocrine group** as more patients are evaluable at ten and fifteen years (Figure 2).

Other authors have also reported improved time to progression and progression-free survival in patients treated by radical prostatectomy and early adjuvant hormonal treatment.

Although there is now clinical and laboratory data suggesting that early endocrine deprivation may offer advantages in progression-free survival of early metastatic prostate cancer, the benefit of radical prostatectomy is less certain. Zincke in 1987 reported on 86 patients with N+ disease who received lymphadenectomy and early hormonal deprivation without prostate removal. When compared to the patients receiving prostatectomy and early deprivation, they did much worse. There are, however, too few patients at risk at five and ten years to make valid conclusions. *More studies are needed to evaluate the benefit of prostatectomy when using early hormonal deprivation.*

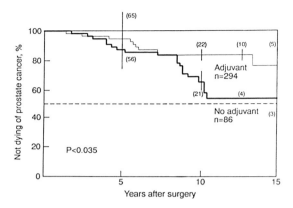

Figure 2. Cause-specific survival in 380 patients with stage N+ (D1) adenocarcinoma of the prostate according to whether or not they received early adjuvant hormonal deprivation (From Zincke H) with permission.

VI. INFLUENCE OF DNA PLOIDY IN STAGE N+ DISEASE

Grade and stage of prostate adenocarcinoma may frequently predict occult nodal metastasis; however, once the lymph nodes are involved, these variables have limited prognostic significance. In order to assist in the allocation of treatment options, better means to stratify patients are necessary. **DNA ploidy analysis is emerging as a potentially accurate means to provide this prognostic information.**

Myers and coworkers retrospectively analyzed the clinical course of 62 patients with stage N+ cancer. All patients were treated with radical prostatectomy and had paraffin-embedded tissue available for retrospective ploidy determination. The patients had a minimum of 9.8 years follow-up and were separated according to DNA histograms and whether they received early (EET) versus delayed (DET) endocrine treatment. Twenty-three patients (37%) had diploid tumors and, of these, 14 received adjuvant early endocrine suppression. No patient with a diploid tumor receiving EET died of prostate cancer and 71% were alive with no evidence of disease (NED). The remaining four patients died of other causes. If patients had nondiploid tumors or did not receive adjuvant endocrine suppression, they faired more poorly. Of 48 patients in the nondiploid or DET groups, only 11(23%) were alive NED and 19 (40%) had died of prostate cancer. Therefore, ploidy was an accurate predictor of clinical outcome and those patients with diploid tumors receiving EET did significantly better than the rest.

Other studies have reviewed the use of DNA ploidy in stage N+ disease and clearly ploidy is superior to other tumor variables in predicting outcome of these patients. The nondiploid tumors progress sooner and are more lethal than their diploid counterparts. *Thus far, no combination of treatment modalities has effectively controlled the nondiploid tumors*. These cases should certainly be considered for aggressive systemic therapeutic protocols.

VII. DISCUSSION

The optimal treatment of patients with stage N+ prostate cancer has not been established. A growing body of retrospective data suggest that, in those patients with diploid tumors, radical prostatectomy combined with early hormonal deprivation, *may prolong time to progression* and *extend disease-free survival*.

The effect of early hormonal deprivation without prostatectomy has shown similar benefit but has not been adequately studied.

No statistical advantages in regard to *long-term survival* have been documented with any of the treatment modalities reported. Therefore, an alternative goal in regard to treatment of stage N+ prostate cancer is *improved quality of life*. Certainly some men will be spared complications associated with local progression by including prostatectomy in the treatment of their advanced prostate cancer. However, the problems of administering aggressive surgical treatment with its associated morbidity and expense to patients when benefit is unproven are obvious.

It is worthy of note that *only 23% of stage N+ (D1) patients treated "expectantly" have local progression requiring surgery*, ie: if all patients had *total prostatectomy* to spare "complications associated with local progression", *77% would not need it.*

Although promising, until survival advantages can be clearly demonstrated, the purported merit of combination surgery / endocrine treatment will continue to be critically compared to patient morbidity and cost. *Awaiting controlled prospective multi-institutional trials, the unbiased endorsement of one treatment over another in stage N+ prostate cancer must be reserved.*

DOCUMENTATION

BYAR D.P., CORLE D.K., Hormone therapy for prostate cancer : Results of the Veterans Administration Cooperative research group studies. NCI Monogr. 1988, 7 : 165.

DEVERE WHITE R.D., BABAIAN R.K., KRIKORIAN J et al : Adjuvant chemotherapy for stage D1 adenocarcinoma of the prostate. Urology 1983, 21 : 270.

PAULSON DF., The prognostic role of lymphadenectomy in adenocarcinoma of the prostate. Urol Clinics North Am 1980; 7:625.

SCHMIDT J.D., GIBBONS R.P., MURPHY G.P. et al : Adjuvant therapy for localized prostate cancer : Results of national prostatic cancer project (NPCP) protocols 900 and 1,000. J. Urol. 1990, 143 : 222A.

ZINCKE H., Combined surgery and immediate adjuvant hormonal treatment for stage D1 adenocarcinoma of the prostate: Mayo clinic experience . seminars in Urol. 1990; 8: 175-183

Conclusion:
Radical Surgery for Advanced Prostate Cancer and for Radiation Failures

William J. Catalona

Division of Urologic Surgery, Washington University Medical Center St. Louis, Missouri, USA

During the last decade *improvements in surgical techniques* have resulted in a dramatic reduction in blood loss and in the incidence of urinary incontinence, impotence and rectal injury associated with radical prostatectomy. These advances, along with the development of *improved methods of detecting radiation failures*, including measurement of serum prostate specific antigen (PSA) levels, prostatic ultrasonography and automatic biopsy guns, have led to a *substantial shift towards surgical treatment of nearly all stages of prostate cancer.*

It was not so long ago that the accepted dogma was that only patients with small clinical stage B tumors were legitimate candidates for radical prostatectomy. Now, urologists at some of our most prestigious institutions recommend radical prostatectomy for patients with stages A, B, C and D1 disease, as well as for those who have failed radiation therapy.

"Neoadjuvant hormonal therapy" or *"endocrine downstaging"* is also commonly used for patients with bulky, clinically localized tumors and for those with extracapsular disease in hopes of enhancing the chances for subsequent complete tumor resection.

Cystoprostatectomy or *total pelvic exenteration* is being performed more frequently for advanced disease and in radiation failures. This aggressive surgical approach is becoming so commonplace that soon it may be accepted as a "community standard" option that must be offered to all patients.

There is *no convincing evidence* that these expanded indications for radical surgery for prostate cancer are justified. *Why have they been so readily embraced by our profession?*

a) One reason is that there are no other potentially curative treatment options for these unfortunate patients.

b) Another is that we have become proficient at performing these operations.

c) Moreover, as surgeons, we want to make every reasonable effort to remove all of the cancer.

However, *are these efforts "reasonable,"* and do we accomplish anything other than providing an element of false hope and postponing the inevitable acceptance of the reality of the situation?

It is my opinion (some may disagree) that we should not recommend radical cancer operations for most patients with stage C or DI disease or for those who have failed radiation therapy.

1. *The case against radical surgery for stage C disease* is that:

a) *Complete tumor excision is almost never achieved* and there is no evidence that adjuvant hormonal or radiation therapy prolongs survival.

b) Most evidence suggests that **adequate local tumor control** can be achieved in the vast majority of cases with the judicious use of radiation therapy, hormonal therapy and transurethral resection. It is questionable whether it is justified to perform a radical cancer operation on all patients to spare the small proportion who will have local problems not controlled by conservative means. Most of the reports, such as that by Kennedy et al., do not support the efficacy of endocrine downstaging.

2. The case against radical prostatectomy in patients with lymph node metastasis is based on the preponderance of published data showing that adjuvant radiation therapy adds little, if anything, to survival in patients with lymph node metastases, and that while adjuvant hormonal therapy may delay cancer progression, it does not prolong survival. The latest update of the Mayo Clinic experience by Myers et al provides no convincing evidence for any greater benefit. Their claim that patients with diploid cancers treated with radical surgery and early endocrine therapy did better than similar patients treated without early endocrine therapy may be viewed skeptically by some biostatisticians as a possible example of "post hoc subset analysis" (dividing the data set into subsets increases the possibility that a "significant" difference will be found between subsets by chance alone).

Moreover, their data still **do not answer the question about how the patients would have done with early endocrine therapy without the radical surgery**. Most published evidence suggests that about 30% of the patients with nodal metastases treated conservatively with hormonal therapy will require transurethral resection for local disease. Thus, the routine performance of radical prostatectomy in all patients with nodal metastases to prevent later local problems trades the morbidity of

transurethral resection in 30% of the patients for that of radical prostatectomy in 100%. Although we have become more proficient at this operation, there is a finite incidence of postoperative complications even in the best of hands (Frazier et al, Borland and Walsh, Zincke, Leandri et al, and Ahlering et al), and this does not appear to be a reasonable trade-off unless the surgeon has extraordinary expertise with the operation and demonstrated low operative morbidity and mortality rates.

3. The case against salvage radical prostatectomy in radiation failures is as follows.

a) *The morbidity of salvage radical prostatectomy is high*. Approximately 10% of the patients will have rectal injuries that will require colostomy for repair, as suggested by Borland and Walsh. Between 10 and 64% of the patients will have postoperative urinary incontinence. Only about 30% of the patients will have pathologically specimen confined cancer with undetectable postoperative PSA levels. These complications and results are documented in the studies by Ahlering et al and by Zincke.

b) Furthermore, **node dissections are difficult** or impossible to perform following radiation therapy.

Taken together, the proportion of patients who have no rectal injury, normal postoperative continence and complete tumor resection with undetectable postoperative PSA levels (without adjuvant hormonal therapy) is only about 15 to 20% as reported by Ahlering et al. These poor prospects for an overall favorable result mitigate against recommending salvage radical prostatectomy in most patients.

c) The performance of **cystoprostatectomy** or **pelvic exenteration** eliminates the risk of urinary incontinence but, as suggested by Zincke, it does not usually allow for complete tumor excision. These extensive operations also carry a substantial risk for postoperative morbidity and impose functional sacrifices in terms of the ileal conduit or continent urinary diversion.

There is no convincing evidence that the benefits of radical surgery offset the associated risks in patients with advanced prostate cancer or in those who have failed radiation therapy. *The available evidence suggests that hormonal therapy alone provides equivalent therapeutic benefits with less potential for morbidity.*

DOCUMENTATION

BORLAND R.N., WALSH P.C. The management of rectal injury during radical retropubic prostatectomy. J. Urol., 147, 905-907, 1992.

FISHER, R. E. AND KOCH, M. O.: Recognition and management of delayed disruption vesicourethral anastomosis in radical prostatectomy. J. Urol., in press.

FRAZIER H.A., ROBERTSON J.E., PAULSON D.F. Radical prostatectomy: the pros and cons of the perineal versus retropubic approach. J. Urol., 147, 888-890, 1992.

LEANDRI P., ROSSIGNOL G., GAUTIER J.R., RAMON J. Radical retropubic prostatectomy: morbidity and quality of life experience with 620 consecutive cases. J. Urol, 147, 883-887, 1992.

MYERS R.P., LARSON-KELLER J.J., BERGSTRALH E.J., ZINCKE H., OESTERLING J.E., LIEBER M.M. Hormonal treatment at time of radical retropubic prostatectomy for stage D1 prostate cancer: Results of long-term follow-up. J. Urol. 147, 910-915, 1992.

ZINCKE H. Radical prostatectomy and extenterative procedures for local failure after radiotherapy with curative intent: comparison of outcomes. J. Urol., 147, 894-899, 1992.

VI

LOCALLY ADVANCED AND METASTATIC DISEASE

Previously Untreated Locally Advanced and Metastatic Prostatic Cancer

S. Khoury

Department of Urology, Hôpital de la Pitié, Paris, France

A management plan can be defined on the basis of the *previous chapters*.

The primary treatment of advanced metastatic prostatic cancers is **mainly hormonal.**

I. WHICH HORMONE THERAPY?

The basic treatment consists of **castration** (either**surgical** or, more and more, chemical by means of **LHRH analogues**).

Should an antiandrogen be associated with castration on a long term basis (maximal androgen blockade)? The results of the literature are conflicting and the conclusions of a meta-analysis study are awaited to show if survival and/or quality of life is enhanced by the initiation of this combined treatment.

II. WHEN SHOULD TREATMENT BE COMMENCED?

The answer depends on the severity of the symptoms presented by the patient :

1. PATIENTS WITH DISTURBING SYMPTOMS

This group represents the majority of patients with metastatic prostatic cancer. They present with symptoms either due to **obstruction** or **secondary to metastases**, particularly bone metastases. **These patients should be treated immediately** after esta-

blishing the diagnosis. 70% of patients respond objectively (reduction in prostatic mass, improvement in metastatic images) and 80% respond subjectively (improvement in obstructive symptoms and metastatic pain, improvement in general status).

a) Bladder neck obstruction

In these cases it is preferable not to perform TUR immediately, as this procedure is frequently superfluous in view of the fact that micturition is improved in the majority of patients by hormonal treatment alone.

Moreover, some authors believe that TUR may contribute to dissemination of the disease. Although there is no objective evidence for this hypothesis, it is nevertheless a general rule in oncology to avoid cutting into the tumour whenever possible.

When **acute urinary retention** is the first presenting symptom of a prostatic tumour, the **bladder is drained** (by suprapubic or transurethral catheter) and a **biopsy is performed**.

Some clinicians prefer to perform a TUR immediately to relieve obstruction. Others prefer not to perform TUR immediately. When histological confirmation is obtained, **hormone treatment** is commenced. Urinary drainage is maintained for 3 to 4 weeks until hormone treatment becomes effective. The majority of patients regain micturition after this period and the catheter can then be permanently removed.

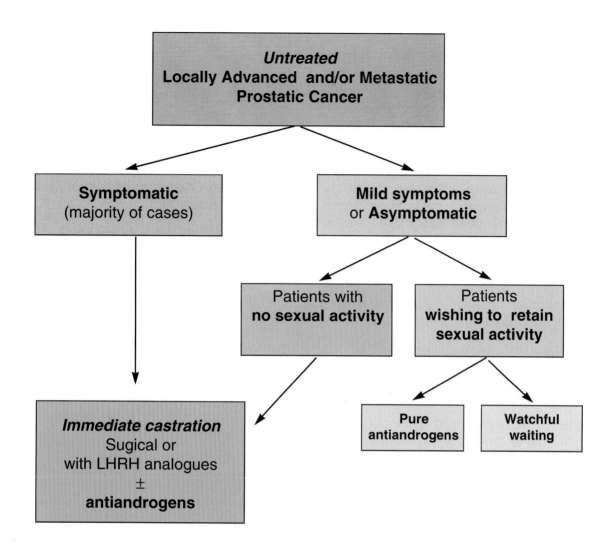

Management of *untreated* metastatic prostate cancer

If micturition is not restored after four weeks despite hormone treatment, **TUR** may be performed.

b) Ureteric obstructive symptoms

A previously untreated patient who presents with oliguria or anuria, or with progressive hydronephrosis and/or renal failure should be offered **hormonal therapy**.

Because an immediate androgen ablation is necessary, it is preferable not to start the treatment with LHRH analogues even associated with an antiandrogen unless the obstructed ureters are stented. **Surgical castration** is preferable in these rare cases.

Ketoconazole also has a very prompt effect and brings testosterone to castrate levels in 24 hours, and therefore can be used to achieve rapid relief of ureteric obstruction, while being reversible at the cessation of treatment.

If acute ureteric obstruction is the **presen-**

ting symptom of a prostatic tumour, castration cannot be performed before histological confirmation of cancer, which may take several days, hormone treatment is commenced by administration of *oestrogens*. This constitutes one of the remaining indications for the use of oestrogens in prostatic cancer.

As a *second step*, hormonal treatment can be continued with surgical castration or LH-RH analogues associated with a short course of antiandrogens to prevent flare-up.

A *temporary nephrostomy* or *internal stenting* might be necessary until the maximum benefit from the hormonal therapy is achieved.

c) Painful bony metastases

Hormonal therapy is the basic treatment.

2. PATIENTS WITH
FEW OR NO SYMPTOMS

a) Patients who no longer have any sexual activity

With new hormone treatment modalities now available, the wait-and-see approach might be prejudicial in terms of survival and quality of survival especially in poor risk patients. Furthermore, it requires much closer surveillance than if treatment is commenced. The risk of this approach is that the patient may develop silent metastases in sensitive points such as the spine or proximal femur with the possibility of pathological fractures with all their consequences. Hormone therapy delays the time to progression of progression of the tumour and improves the quality of the patient's life. For all of these reasons, it seems preferable, in patients with no sexual activity, to *commence hormone therapy immediately after the diagnosis*.

b) Patients who wish to retain sexual activity

In sexually active patients who wish to retain this activity, it is legitimate to *withhold hormone treatment* and simply observe the patient. These patients are also an indication for *pure antiandrogens* which do not present a major effect on sexual activity.

3. What is the duration of response to hormone therapy ?

Unfortunately, the clinical response to hormone treatment only lasts an average of 2-3 years. After this period of time, if the patient has not died from another cause, which is frequently the case in prostatic cancer, recurrence is inevitable and the phase of hormone resistance begins. The therapeutic possibilities at this stage become much more problematic and require good coordination so that the side effects of the various modalities do not cancel out the frequently limited benefit which can be obtained from them.

DOCUMENTATION

DENIS L. Current strategies in hormonal manipulation of advanced prostate cancer. Current Opinion in urology 1991, 1:16-20.

MCCONNEL J.D. Physiologic basis of endocrine therapy for prostate cancer, Urol Clinic North Am 1991, 18, N°1, 1-14.

Management of Hormone-Escaped Prostatic Cancer

S. Khoury

Clinique Urologique, Hôpital de la Pitié, Paris, France

I. DEFINITION

Although the majority of patients (70%) with prostatic cancer respond objectively and/or subjectively to hormone treatment, an escape phenomenon occurs after an average of 2 to 3 years

Hormone-resistant stage T3 or M+ prostatic cancer is defined by the fact that the disease continues to progress despite a well conducted hormone treatment.

Non-compliance with the treatment regimen (often seen in elderly men) should be ruled out, by the observation of castrate level serum testosterone, as the main reason for treatment failure.

This escape results from selection of preexisting or *de novo* appearance of hormone resistant clones

What is the definition of progression?

Classically, definition of failure of the primary treatment and progression was based on clinical criteria. Now that PSA has been shown to be a good marker of tumour progression, we have to consider that the primary treatment has failed as soon as PSA starts to rise again. These biological changes precede the clinical progression by several months .

II. SECOND LINE HORMONAL TREATMENT

1. When should a second line hormonal treatment be considered ?

An alternative treatment must be considered when the level of **PSA starts rising**, when **new spots appear** on follow-up bone scan and of course when the patient becomes **symptomatic again**. The more we wait the less effective will be the second line hormone therapy.

2. When a cancer is resistant to a primary hormonal treatment can it still respond to another hormonal treatment ?

At present there are no generally accepted rules for second line endocrine management. The varying sets of parameters and criteria used by different groups of investigators in order to evaluate response, make comparisons of widely different therapeutic regimens very difficult.

We know already that our capacity to prolong survival is limited and this means that our choice for second line therapy should aim more at improving the quality than the duration of survival, taking into consideration the patient's specific expectations and wishes.

Which endocrine therapy to choose is determined by factors which are dependent on the patient, the tumour and the first line therapy.

In practice we are mainly faced with two situations

a) Can a cancer resistant to castration, for example, respond to oestrogens and vice versa?

When the patient has been castrated and relapses, a subjective response can be obtained in some cases by using **high doses of oestrogens**. If the patient was already receiving oestrogens, castration only exceptionally induces remission.

b) Can a cancer resistant to surgical or chemical castration (oestrogens or LHRH agonist) still respond to antiandrogens?

Despite the contradictory results reported in the literature, everyday experience shows that antiandrogens appear to be inactive in the presence of resistance to standard hormone treatment.

3. Are there any other effective hormonal modalities.

New hormonal treatments have been developed lately. The results have been disappointing due in particular to important side effects. A review is included in another chapter of this book.

4. In the case of true hormone escape, should we stop hormonal treatment?

The answer is that the treatment **should not be stopped**, as a hormone refractory tumour is heterogeneous and still contains androgen-dependent cells. This is demonstrated by the flare-up obtained with the administration of testosterone to such patients.

II. ALTERNATIVE TREATMENTS OTHER THAN HORMONES

1. What are the treatment options after true hormonal treatment failure ?

At this stage treatment becomes difficult and results are poor. The alternatives include :

a) Chemotherapy

b) Radiotherapy

2. Rationale of treatment

a) Characteristics of hormone-resistant cases

♦ **1)** The hormone-resistant stage of prostatic cancer is the **most advanced stage** of the disease.

♦ **2)** The mean **survival** is generally less than 1 year.

♦ **3)** There is **no curative treatment** at this stage.

b) Presenting clinical features

At this stage, the patient presents with either :

♦ **1) Obstructive urinary symptoms** due to local progression of the tumour : dysuria, infection, hydronephrosis, etc.

♦ 2) or **symptoms due to metastases** (particularly bone metastases), in the form of osteoarticular pain, deterioration in the general status and reduced performance status.

♦ 3) A **combination** of these two manifestations.

c) Basis of the treatment strategy

As treatment is therefore **purely palliative**, it is essential to :

♦ 1) **start with the least toxic** and best tolerated treatments;

◆ 2) **follow a stepped protocol** depending on the patient's symptoms and general status, keeping in mind that survival is not the only objective, but that quality of survival is also important ;

◆ 3) in the practical management of the patient, **dissociate** therapeutic approaches adopted in the context of a **research protocol,** the efficacy of which has yet to be demonstrated, from those **treatments with proven efficacy.** Only these latter modalities should be considered when an individual patient is treated in isolation, in the absence of any therapeutic research protocol.

As **treatment is symptomatic** in nature, it varies depending on whether it is designed to treat **obstructuve urinary symptoms** or **symptoms secondary to metastases**.

III. MANAGEMENT OF URINARY TRACT OBSTRUCTION

1. Management of bladder outlet obstruction

◆ Obstruction is *severe*

a) TUR

The aim of TUR is to mechanically remove the obstruction of the bladder neck by the prostatic tumour.

◆ 1) *Should the resection consist of making a simple tunnel or should as much of the tumour mass as possible be removed?*

A recent study has shown that it is better to resect as extensively as possible, as the risk of incontinence does not appear to be appreciably increased. This avoids early recurrences which are fairly frequent when a simple tunnel is made. However, in both cases, the risk of postoperative incontinence is not negligible (3 - 4%).

◆ 2) *Should this TUR be associated with radiotherapy or palliative chemotherapy to prevent rapid recurrence of obstruction ?*

The value of this adjuvant treatment has not been demonstrated. In 30 to 40% of cases, however, **radiotherapy appears to delay recurrence** of the obstruction (Bagshaw). Patients with an urethral catheter must not be irradiated. If the patient has signs of obstruction, TUR must be performed first, if at all possible. Otherwise, a cystostomy catheter must be inserted prior to radiotherapy.

◆ Obstruction is *moderate*

a) Estramustine phosphate (Estracyt®)

This treatment symptomatically improves one out of three patients for a mean duration of 4 months. The advantage of this treatment is that it is prescribed on an outpatient basis and is not associated with any major toxicity. These results are certainly modest, but it must be remembered that from the time the patient becomes hormone-resistant, the therapeutic modalities available are very limited and, most importantly, they are all associated with side effects which, in some cases, are severe.

If no result is obtained with Estracyt® after 3 to 4 weeks or if the patient becomes resistant after an initial phase of response, we proceed to TUR

2. Management of ureteric obstruction

a) What can be done when the patient presents with anuria ?

Anuria is generally due to obstruction of the ureters by **invasion of the trigone** by the tumour. In some cases it may be due to extrinsic **compression** of the lumbar ureter by enlarged para-aortic lymph nodes and in some to **non-neoplastic causes** (obstruction of a single functioning kidney by uric acid stones, ...)

◆ **1)** The first step is to **treat the water and electrolyte disorders of** these patients and administer high doses of cortisone (200 mg of hydrocortisone twice a day). A **percutaneous nephrostomy** is inserted.

◆ **2)** The next step is **antegrade or retrograde insertion of a bilateral indwelling double J stent**. In many cases this is not possible due to deformation of the trigone. Consequently, these cases are best treated first by **deep resection of the trigone** and then by antegrade or retrograde insertion of an internal diversion double J stent.

◆ **3)** When the **patency of the ureter cannot be restored** either leave a nephrostomy tube in place (short life expetancy) or perform bilateral cutaneous ureterostomy (longer life expectancy).

IV. MANAGEMENT OF METASTASES

In practice, these patients suffer from their **bone metastases** (the other metastases occur much later in the course of the disease and are often less important clinically).

We shall not discuss **painless metastases** which do not require any particular treatment apart from that of the primary tumour. However spine and hips must be watched for possible pathological fractures

In the case of **painful metastases**, treatment depends on whether these metastases are **localized** or **disseminated**.

The therapeutic response is determined by evaluating the quantity and the type of the analgesics required by the patient and the performance status (Karnofsky, WHO).

1. Localized symptomatic metastases

In the case of a localized metastasis with pain directly related to the lesion, the best treatment remains **local radiotherapy** to the site of the metastasis. This radiotherapy should be of low intensity. Local radiotherapy can relieve pain in 80% of cases. This analgesia lasts several months and more than a year in 60% of responders who survive beyond this period.

In the event of **recurrence of the pain**, further irradiation is generally ineffective.

When localized metastases fail to respond to radiotherapy, the management is the same as that for disseminated lesions.

2. Disseminated symptomatic metastases

In the presence of disseminated metastatic lesions, when the **pain is not associated with one particular lesion**, treatment should follow a stepped protocol.

a) We first put the patient on non-specific analgesics (anti-inflammatory agents are particularily effective. **Estramustine phosphate** is then given (4 capsules per day for 3 weeks or 1 month). One patient out of 3 obtains significant remission of pain (enabling to stop or greatly reduce analgesics) for an average of 3 to 4 months.

If the patient does not respond or no longer responds to estramustine phosphate, classical chemotherapy must be prescribed.

b) Chemotherapy

None of the agents used are particularly active ; the objective response rates are about 10%. Consequently, the best tolerated drugs should be used. Various clinical trials have also shown that there is no advantage in combining several drugs, as the toxicity is increased without any gain in activity.

We have continued to use **cyclophospha-mide** by infusion at a dose of 500 mg per day in monthly cycles of 3 to 4 days depending on the general status. This treatment achieves substantial improvement in pain in 30% of cases, but unfortunately, this effect only lasts for an average of three or four months.

Vincristine + estramustine phosphate seems to give better results than either of these 2 drugs alone (H. Scher).

Infusion of **high doses of tetrasodium fos-festerol** (1.5 g per day) also gives appreciable results on pain.

c) Role of radiotherapy

The action of radiotherapy, which is a local treatment, is limited in the case of disseminated lesions and when the origin of the pain is difficult to determine. **Large field irradiation** has been attempted and has occasionally given results when the region responsible for the pain has been included in the field of irradiation.

Some authors have proposed **half-body irradiation**, particularly of the lower half of the body, which is the most frequent site of pain. Patients treated by this method are generally at the terminal stage of the disease. **Analgesia has been achieved in a large number of cases**, but it is difficult to evaluate the duration, as these patients often die soon after this irradiation probably because of their already severely impaired general status.

d) Are *isotopes* such as phosphorus or strontium indicated in the treatment of painful metastases ?

Certain radioactive isotopes, such as phosphorus or strontium, have a special affinity for bone and bone metastases. The use of **radioactive phosphorus** has been abandoned as this product has a very penetrating γ emission which causes sclerosis of

vessels and bone marrow, inducing marrow aplasia. More recently, **radioactive strontium**, which has an isotope emitting β radiation, has been used. Because of its poor penetration it respects the vessels at the periphery of the tumour and does not necessitate isolation of the patient. Spectacular results have occasionally been published in the literature. In a study which we conducted in twenty patients in collaboration with Prof. Ancri at the Hôpital de la Pitié, in Paris, radioactive strontium unfortunately did not demonstrate sufficient activity to justify the manipulation and use of this radioactive isotope with a relatively long half-life (56 days) with all of the risks and disadvantages which that involves for the environment. Fossä was also unable to confirm the good results reported in the literature.

e) What is left at this stage after all of the semi-specific modalities have been tried?

We are left with **non-specific analgesia,** which has progressed considerably over recent years. The treatment of a patient with advanced disseminated metastases involves the simultaneous administration of high doses of morphine and high doses of non-steroidal, then steroidal anti-inflammatory agents. Regular three to four week courses of calcitonin constitute a valuable adjuvant. Chlodronate and pamidronate, antihypercalcaemic agents, are excellent analgesics for multiple bone pain. Treatment is started via the intravenous route for 3 to 4 days and is then continued orally for as long as necessary. These drugs are not hypocalcaemic when the serum calcium level is normal.

As a result of these advances, **pain can be controlled in the majority of patients**. When the patient reaches this stage, the doctor's role is to prevent the patient from suffering and to help him to retain a certain dignity. This is the first priority.

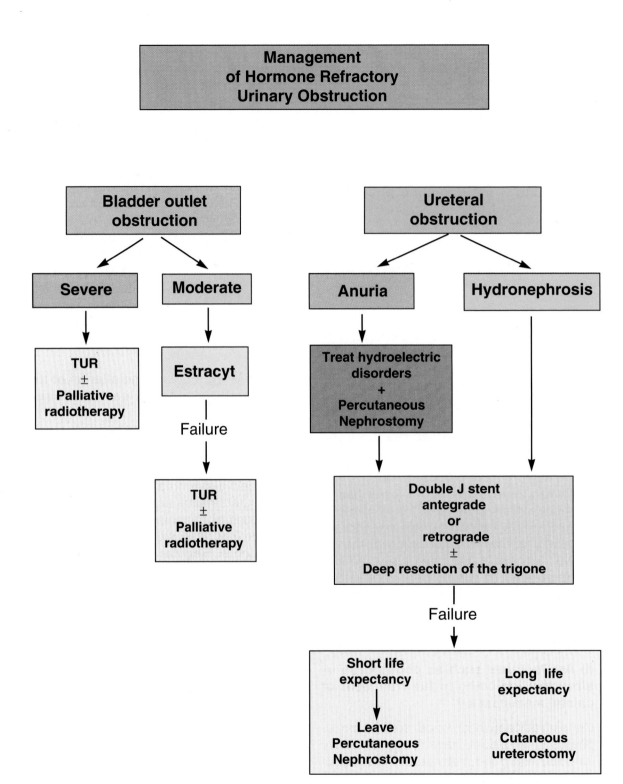

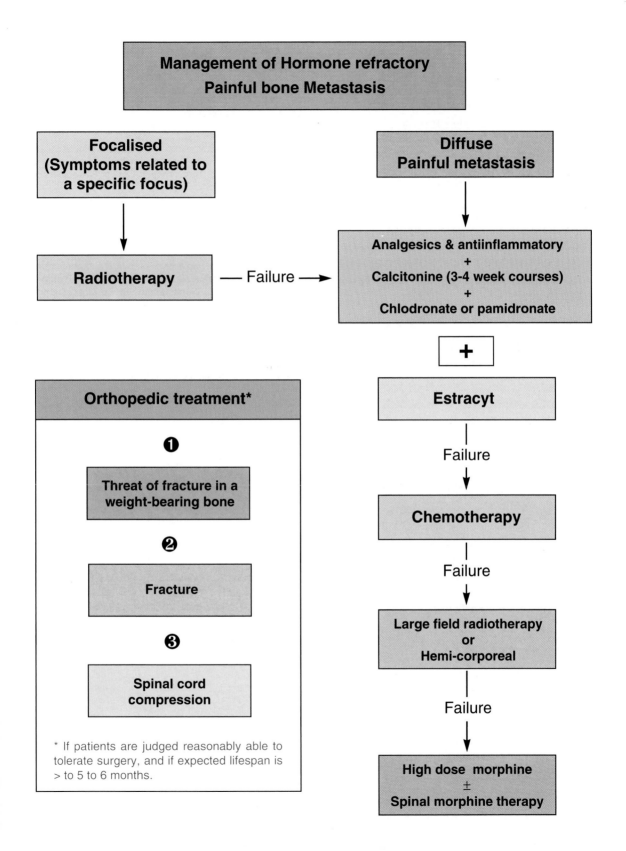

V. SPECIFIC CASES

1. Spinal cord compression

The treatment of spinal cord compression secondary to metastatic prostate cancer is palliative. An important goal is to prevent the condition. When it occurs, however, the goals are to reverse the neurologic deficit, relieve the pain, and improve the quality of life for the patient. (see special article page 213).

High-dose steroids (dexamethasone) should be instituted immediately, and endocrine therapy should be started if not already in use.

a) Ambulatory and moderately paraparetic patients seem best treated initially with radiation alone. Immediate surgical decompression should be used in patients with an expected lifespan of at least 6 months who deteriorate during radiation, who have had previous radiation to the involved site, or who have a potentially correctable unstable spine.

b) Paraplegic patients or severely paraparetic patients with recent neurologic deterioration should be treated with immediate surgical decompression if they are judged reasonably able to tolerate the surgery. These patients should then receive post-operative radiation treatment.

2. Orthopaedic treatment

Orthopaedic treatment is indicated in bone metastases when there is :

a) a *threat of fracture* **in a weight-bearing bone** (hip, vertebrae ...).or

b) a *fracture*

Stabilisation of the spine requires the use of posterior plates screwed into the pedicles of the vertebrae.

These orthopaedic procedures are obviously only indicated when the patient has an appreciable life expectancy, generally greater than 3 months.

DOCUMENTATION

EMRICH L.J., PRIORE R.L., MURPHY G.P., BRADY M.F., and the investigators of the national prostatic cancer project (1985). Prognostic factors in patients with advanced stage prostate cancer. Cancer Research 45 : 5173-5179.

GIBBONS R.P. (1981). Investigators, National Cancer Project Cooperative Clinical Trials. Cooperative clinical trials of single and combined agent protocols : Adjuvant protocols. Urology 17 (suppl) : 48-52.

ISAACS J.T. (1985). New principles in the management of metastatic prostate cancer. In Schroeder F., Richards B. (eds) : "EORTC Genitourinary Group Monograph 2, Part A : Therapeutic Principles in Metastatic Prostate Cancer, "New York : Alan R. Liss, pp 383-405.

SCHIPPER H., CLINCH J., MCMURRAY A., LEVITT M. (1984). Measuring the quality of life of cancer patients : The functional living index-cancer : Development and validation. J. Clin. Oncol. 2 : 472-483.

Management of Patients with Spinal Cord Compression Secondary to Metastatic Prostatic Carcinoma

Daniel F. Flynn and William U. Shipley

Department of Radiation Medicine, Massachusetts General Hospital Cancer Center;
Harvard Medical School, Boston, Massachusetts

The treatment of spinal cord compression secondary to metastatic prostate cancer is palliative. An important goal is to prevent the condition. When it occurs nevertheless, the goals are to reverse the neurologic deficit, relieve the pain, and improve the quality of life for the patient.

I. MECHANISM

In metastatic prostatic cancer, the extradural (epidural) space of the spinal cord is involved, most commonly, secondarily by **extension from an eroded vertebral body** arch or spinous process. There may also be an element of compression secondary to the **collapse and displacement of a bony element**. Significant vertebral body collapse, especially with angulation of the spine, appears to make the prognosis for recovery less favorable (Table 1).

II. CLINICAL PRESENTATION

Spinal cord compression secondary to prostate cancer is more apt to occur in patients who present initially with **advanced stage** disease and **poorly differentiated** tumors.

The high likelihood of bone metastases from prostatic cancer is well recognized. To diagnose cord or cauda equina compression early in these patients, **a high index of suspicion must be maintained** for the typical signs and symptoms.

As with metastases from other primary sites, **pain** is the dominant initial symptom.

Weakness, **sensory deficit**, and **autonomic dysfunction** usually occur later.

In two series on prostatic cancer cord compression by Shoskes and Perrin and Iacovov and coworkers, back pain was the initial symptom in 75% and 92%, respectively.

In the Massachusetts General Hospital series, 14 of the 56 patients (25%) had spinal cord compression as the **initial presentation** of malignancy. This was the case in 11 of the 37 patients (29%) in the series of Iacovov and associates and 5 of the 14 patients (36%) in the series of Liskow and coworkers. All patients in our series had an abnormal prostate gland palpated on rectal examination, with an elevated serum acid phosphatase in all but one case. In the series by Iacovov et al, the serum acid phosphatase was elevated in all 26 cases in which it was measured.

The **location of the compression** is most often the thoracic spine, as it is with other primary malignancies, with an average of 67% for prostatic cancer. In our series of 56 patients with 69 sites of spinal cord compression, the thoracic spine was involved 73% of the time.

All clinicians should consider cord compression as a **possibility** in any patient with prostatic cancer and back pain. All patients with known osseous metastases should be advised by their clinicians to **seek medical care** within hours should they develop leg weakness. With the use of serial evaluations (including a serum prostate-specific antigen assay) during follow-up visits, such unanticipated progressions of disease will be less frequent.

III. DIAGNOSTIC RADIOLOGIC STUDIES

Today MRI is the primary diagnostic tool for spinal cord or cauda equina compression. Emergency myelography is reserved for those patients who cannot undergo a technically adequate or expeditious MRI procedure.

An MRI scan of the entire spine is necessary as multiple sites of compression are common (23%) and a regional MRI centered on the supect area may fail to detect the other compression sites

IV. TREATMENT PRINCIPLES

Because patients with spinal cord or cauda equina compression from metastatic disease are not curable, **palliation is the goal of treatment**. Preservation or restoration of ambulation and bladder function are the measures of successful treatment. Pain relief is also an important goal.

1. Medical treatment

a) Corticosteroids have been reported to be of benefit in reducing neurologic deficit. The optimum dose in humans with spinal cord compression has not been established. A dose of dexamethasone (Decadron) of 10 mg intravenously followed by 4 mg orally every 6 hours is commonly used. Some authors have recommended higher doses.

Table1. Number of patients with spinal cord compression from metastatic prostatic cancer, by clinical stage and tumor differentiation.

Stage at diagnosis	TUMOR DIFFERENTIATION			
	Well	Moderate	Poor	Totals (%)
T2 (B)	0	0	3	3/207 (1,4)
T3-T4 (C)	0	4	7	11/197 (5,6)
M1 (D2)	5	4	18	27/157 (17,2)
Total	5/175	8/191	28/29	41/595 (6,8)

Data from Kuban Da, El-Mahdi AM, Sigfred SV, et al: Characteristics of spinal cord compression in adenocarcinoma of prostate. Urology 28: 364, 1986.

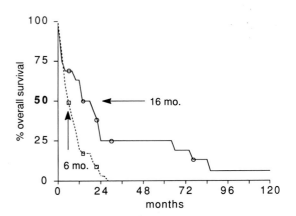

Figure 1. Overall survival after the diagnosis of spinal cord compression from epidural metastatic prostatic cancer in 51 patients treated at our institution. The dashed curve represents the 35 patients who did not respond to (progressed on) endocrine therapy (median survival, 6 months), the solid curve represents the 16 patients whose treatment included the initiation of endocrine therapy (median survival 16 months).

b) Endocrine therapy (androgen deprivation) has an important role in the treatment of spinal cord compression if the patients have not yet received this.

Because an **immediate androgen ablation is necessary**, it is preferable not to start the treatment with LHRH analogs even under the cover of antiandrogens. **Surgical castration** is preferable in these rare cases. If this is not feasible **oestrogens** are an alternative. LHRH analogs could be given later when the neurological problem has been resolved.

◆ Cases with no previous hormonal treatment

In the Massachusetts General Hospital series, of all patients treated with hormones for the first time at the diagnosis of cord compression, 9 of the 16 who were bedridden became ambulatory, including 6 of the 10 patients who were paraplegic.

◆ Hormone resistant cases

For the bedridden patients whose disease had failed endocrine therapy at the time of cord compression, only 12 of 30 became ambulatory, including only 2 of 11 paraplegic patients.

The median survival time for the 16 patients who had endocrine therapy initiated at the diagnosis of cord compression was 16 months compared with 6 months for the 35 patients who had failed endocrine therapy (Figure 1).

2. Surgery and radiotherapy

Treatments of spinal cord compression from prostatic cancer have been surgery only, radiation only, or combined surgery plus radiation.

To better understand the following results, paraplegia was defined as bedridden with complete loss of antigravity movement of one or more extremities. This included cases in which the patient could partially tense the extremity muscles, drag one or both heels slightly, or wiggle the toes. Converting a paraplegic patient to paraparetic status is considered as a partial response.

a) Surgery

In a series of patients treated primarily by surgery, Shoskes and Perrin reported that all ambulatory patients remained ambulatory and 8 of 13 bedridden patients (62%) became ambulatory postoperatively. In a similar surgical series reported by Iacovov et

Table 2. Post-treatment ambulatory rate of bedridden patients with cord compression from prostate cancer.

TREATMENT	NUMBER	PER CENT
Surgery alone	4/11	36
Radiation alone	8/15	53
Surgery plus radiation	8/18	44

Table 3. Post-treatment ambulation in paraplegic patients according to treatment.

TIME PARAPLEGIC (HOURS)	SURGERY	RADIATION	BOTH	TOTAL
Less than 24	1/2	–	3/5	4/7
Between 24 and 72	0/2	2/4	0/1	2/7
Greater than 72	0/2	0/2	1/2	1/6

al, all seven ambulatory patients remained ambulatory and 14 of 27 bedridden patients (52%) became ambulatory postoperatively. In that series, of the 20 patients who could walk after laminectomy, 15 remained ambulatory until death. Of the 18 patients who required urinary catheterization 9 made sufficient recovery to make this unnecessary. Of the entire group of 34 patients who complained of back pain, decompression relieved pain in 26 (77%) sufficiently to stop the narcotic analgesics.

b) Radiotherapy

The best success with treatment by radiation alone was with ambulatory and moderately paraparetic patients, not with paraplegic patients, in whom the results were poor.

Only two of six such patients treated with radiation alone showed improvement, compared with 10 of 14 when surgery was the initial treatment.

c) Surgery + radiotherapy

In the Massachusetts General Hospital series, restoration of ambulation in bedridden patients appeared more likely if the treatment was radiation alone or surgery plus radiation rather than surgery alone (Table 2).

Management of spinal cord compression

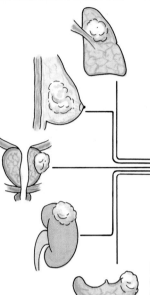

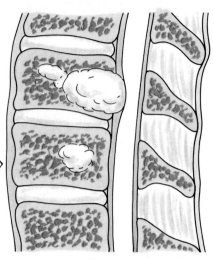

In metastatic prostatic cancer, the extradural (epidural) space of the spinal cord is involved, most commonly, secondarily **by extension** from an eroded vertebral body arch or spinous process. There may also be an element of compression secondary to the **collapse and displacement of a bony element.**

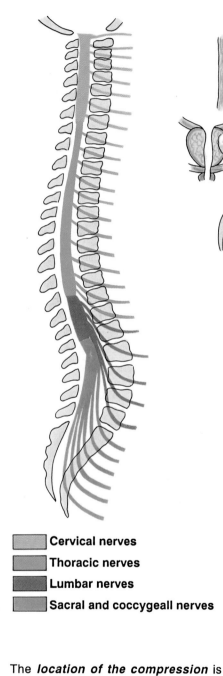

Cervical nerves

Thoracic nerves

Lumbar nerves

Sacral and coccygeall nerves

The **location of the compression** is most often the **thoracic spine,** as it is with other primary malignancies, with an average of 67% for prostatic cancer

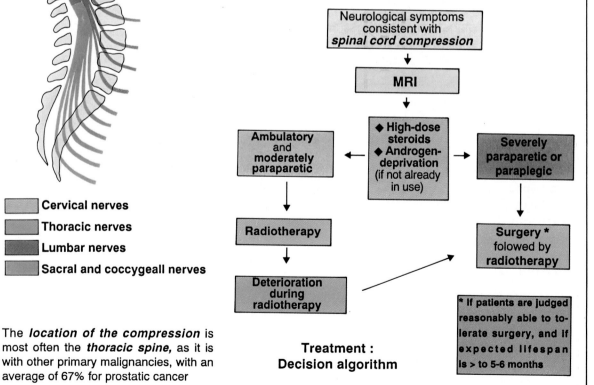

Neurological symptoms consistent with *spinal cord compression*

↓

MRI

↓

◆ **High-dose steroids**
◆ **Androgen-deprivation** (if not already in use)

Ambulatory and moderately paraparetic

↓

Radiotherapy

↓

Deterioration during radiotherapy

Severely paraparetic or paraplegic

↓

Surgery * folowed by **radiotherapy**

* If patients are judged reasonably able to tolerate surgery, and if expected lifespan is > to 5-6 months

Treatment :
Decision algorithm

216

3. Results and complications

In our series, patients were ambulatory after treatment when their pretreatment status was ambulatory (100%), paraparetic (52%), and paraplegic (38%). Our data show that the response to treatment may be a function of the length of time the patient is paraplegic before treatment (Table 3).

In our series, there were 4 (8%) **deaths** among 56 patients less than 30 days after treatment: two treated with radiation and two with surgery. There were four **complications** noted: a pulmonary embolism, a myocardial infarction, an epidural hematoma, and a severe pancytopenia.

4. Survival

In the series of lacovov and associates, 50% of the patients with cord compression by prostatic cancer were alive at 1 year and 30% at 2 years. In the review by Barcena et al, the median survival was 13 months. The median survival of the Massachusetts General Hospital patients was 7 months, with 17 patients (31%) alive at 1 year, 7 patients (13%) alive at 2 years, and 4 patients (7%) alive at 5 years after the diagnosis of cord compression.

Survival is dependent primarily on the **progression of systemic disease** rather than on the localized disease causing cord compression. Significant long-term survival is possible when hormonal manipulation is initiated at the time of cord compression, compared with patients already in relapse after hormonal therapy when they present with cord compression (see Fig. 1).

SUMMARY

Spinal cord or cauda equina compression from prostatic cancer is an oncologic emergency necessitating prompt evaluation and treatment. The strong correlation between pretreatment motor status and treatment outcome underscores the importance of immediate treatment before further neurologic deterioration and before the damage to the spinal cord becomes permanent.

Patients with known osseous metastases should be alerted by their clinicians to seek medical help within hours should they develop weakness in an extremity. Prompt MRI of the entire spine should be done prior to treatment. Myelography should be reserved for those patients who cannot undergo a technically adequate or expeditious MRI study. The convenience of MRI relative to myelography allows clinicians to diagnose actual or impending spinal cord compression earlier.

High-dose steroids (dexamethasone) should be instituted immediately, and endocrine therapy should be started if not already in use.

Ambulatory and moderately paraparetic patients seem best treated initially with radiation alone. Immediate surgical decompression should be used in patients with an expected lifespan of at least 6 months who deteriorate during radiation, who have had previous radiation to the involved site, or who have a potentially correctable unstable spine. In addition, paraplegic patients or severely paraparetic patients with recent neurologic deterioration should be treated with immediate surgical decompression if they are judged reasonably able to tolerate the surgery. These patients should then receive postoperative radiation treatment.

DOCUMENTATION

BARCENA A, LOBATO RD, RIVAS JJ, et al: Spinal metastatic disease: An analysis of factors determining functional prognosis and the choice of treatment. Neurosurgery 15:820-827, 1984

BLACK P: Spinal metastasis: Current status and recommended guidelines for management. Neurosurgery 5:726-746, 1979

BONNER JA, LICHTER AS: A caution about the use of MRI to diagnose spinal cord compression. N Engl J Med 322:556-557, 1990

IACOVOV JW, MARKS JC, ABRAMS PH, et al: Cord compression and carcinoma of the prostate: Is laminectomy justified? Br J Urol 57:733-736, 1985

KUBAN DA, EL-MAHDI AM, SIGFRED SV, et al: Characteristics of spinal cord compression in adenocarcinoma of prostate. Urology 28:364-369, 1986

PERRIN RG, MCBROOM RJ: Anterior versus posterior decompression for symptomatic spinal metastasis. Can J Neurol Sci 14:75-80, 1987

SHOSKES DA, PERRIN RG: The role of surgical management for symptomatic spinal cord compression patients with metastatic prostate cancer. J Urol 142:337-339, 1989

SIEGAL T: Surgical decompression of anterior and posterior malignant epidural tumors compressing the spinal cord: A prospective study. Neurosurgery 17:424-432, 1985

SUNDARESAN N, GALICICH JH, LANE JM, et al: Treatment of neoplastic epidural cord compression by vertebral body resection and stabilization. J Neurosurg 63:676684, 1985

USHIO Y, POSNER R, POSNER JB, et al: Experimental spinal cord compression by epidural neoplasm. Neurology (Minneap) 27:422-429, 1977

Non-Specific Treatments for Prostatic Cancer Pain

Evelyne Pichard-Léandri

Unité de Diagnostic et Traitement de la Douleur Adulte et Enfants, Institut Gustave-Roussy,
Villejuif, France

Pain is one of the predominant symptoms of prostatic cancer. It may be the presenting symptom, it may accompany the progression of the disease or it may become the major symptom in the terminal phase. This pain reflects, with equal frequency, either loco-regional progression (invasion of nerves, vessels, soft tissues) or disseminated bone metastases (highly osteophilic cancer). Pain may sometimes be secondary to specific treatment.

Regardless of the stage of the disease, the *"pain symptom"* should be treated separately (by non-specific treatment). The cancer responsible for the pain should be treated simultaneously for as long as this is possible (specific treatment).

I. DRUG TREATMENTS

1. How to prescribe drugs

◆ By using the *simplest route available*, oral or rectal, which is equally simple and minimally invasive. The subcutaneous route can be used exceptionally or for long-term treatment when there are contraindications or limitations to the use of other routes of administration.

◆ By prescribing and *administering the analgesic indicated regularly* in order to prevent recrudescence of the pain as well as fear or memory of the pain.

◆ By *adapting the choice* of pharmaceutical form to the particular patient.

◆ By *preventing the side effects* inherent to any centrally-acting analgesic.

◆ By *avoiding coprescription* of drugs with the same or similar potency, but by potentiating their effects by using certain adjuvants (anti-inflammatory drugs, psychotropic drugs, etc.).

2. Which drugs should be used ?

The therapeutic protocol is composed of *three different levels* involving the use of analgesics and possibly coanalgesics of increasing potency. The passage from one level to another is determined by failure or inefficacy of the drugs of the previous level when they have been properly prescribed, administered and absorbed.

a) Group I analgesics include *acetylsalicylic acid* and *paracetamol* (4 to 6 grams per day). Glafenine is not an alternative because, while not offering any appreciable superiority, it is associated with considerable risks. *Noramidopyrine* may be proposed in certain circumstances.

The use of the drugs of this first group is frequently short-lived, as they rapidly become ineffective in relation to the severity of the pain. On the other hand, in this category, the non steroidal anti-inflammatory agents (*NSAI*) have a good and lasting efficacy and are particularly suitable for the treatment of bone metastases (Indomethacin, Ibuprofen, Naproxen, Diclofenac, etc.).

b) Group II analgesics are *more potent* than those of the previous group and include *codeine* (in the form of combinations: paracetamol-codeine, aspirin-codeine, sustained-release codeine (Dicodin®) and *dextropropoxyphene* (also available in combinations). *Buprenorphine* (Temgesic®) is administered via the strict sublingual route every 6 or 8 hours. These molecules, although closely resembling true narcotics, are distinguished by their "antagonist" potential and *must never be coprescribed with narcotics* (codeine, dextropropoxyphene, morphine).These drugs are often effective for a fairly long time, but the severity of the pain may require the use of group III drugs.

c) Group III analgesics. This group corresponds to the *narcotics*, represented by *morphine base*. When equi-analgesic doses are used, morphine is equally effective via oral or parenteral administration (10 mg parenterally = 25 to 30 mg orally).

It is initially prescribed in the form of a *potion*. The starting doses are 0.5 to 1 mg/kg/day in six regularly divided doses.

In practice, a 60 kg man will need 5 to 10 mg per dose six times a day (the doses are decreased in the elderly and/or in patients with renal failure).

The mean effective individual dose has been found to be 30 to 40 mg (3 mg/kg/day).

Morphine is available in the form of *sustained-release tablets*. This form has the same efficacy as the potion, but has the advantage of allowing oral doses every twelve hours (instead of every four hours for the potion), relieving the patient and family from the constraints of the dose schedule.

When morphine solution is replaced by sustained-release morphine, the daily dose remains the same : 10 mg of potion every four hours = 60 mg/day = one 30 mg tablet morning and evening. This tablet must not be ground or crushed, as this would induce dangerous massive release of the active ingredient in the proximal segment of the gastrointestinal tract.

Continuous subcutaneous or intravenous administration may be necessary when the oral route cannot be used or when the adverse effects are excessive. The use of a *self-administration continuous infusion pump* improves the quality of the analgesia and frequently decreases the total dose of morphine administered.

d) Coanalgesic drugs

These drugs consist of certain *psychotropics, anticonvulsants, thymoanaleptics and neuroleptics.* They have a potentiating function, but must be prescribed with moderation so as not to increase or add further side effects. Post-radiation or postoperative pain, somatic disafferentation pain and tenesmus respond almost exclusively to combinations of coanalgesics.

II. INVASIVE TREATMENTS

1. The primary invasive treatment is spinal morphine therapy. It is only indicated in the case of failure of traditional drug treatment or unacceptable side effects.

It involves the insertion of a perispinal or intradural catheter, possibly connected, depending on the technique, to a subcutaneous injection site. This system allows the repeated or continuous administration of low doses of morphine (several mg per day).

The lumbar positioning of the catheter ensures relief of pelvic pain.

The administration of drugs other than morphine and the use of sensory nerve root section surgery are exceptional.

2. Cerebroventricular morphine therapy.

This technique is based on the same principle as spinal morphine therapy : application of morphine adjacent to central morphine receptors. It ensures generalised analgesia and may be indicated in the treatment of disseminated metastases when oral and parenteral routes are impossible or ineffective.

III. PARTICULAR CASE OF BONE METASTASES

The treatment of metastatic bone pain follows the same stepped protocol, but *anti-inflammatory agents* are very useful in combination with other drugs, throughout the treatment.

The treatment of a patient with advanced disseminated metastases involves the simultaneous administration of:

◆ high doses of *morphine* and

◆ high doses of *non-steroidal*, then *steroidal anti-inflammatory agents*.

Regular three to four week courses of *calcitonin* constitute a valuable adjuvant.

Chlodronate and *pamidronate*, antihypercalaemic agents, are excellent analgesics for multiple bone pain. Treatment is started via the intravenous route for 3 to 4 days and is then continued orally for as long as necessary. These drugs are not hypocalcaemic when the serum calcium level is normal.

The use of palliative half-body irradiation, localized bone embolisation (spine) and, most importantly, prophylactic or curative orthopaedic surgery with the use of cement for metastatic fractures of weight-bearing segments should also be considered, regardless of the patient's life expectancy.

In conclusion, a simple range of drugs, a rigorous analysis of the pain and a methodical approach can ensure real comfort for these patients, both in terms of pain and autonomy, regardless of the stage of the disease.

DOCUMENTATION

HANKS GW, HOSKIN PJ, AHERNE GW, TURNER P, POULAIN Ph. Explanation for potency of repeated oral doses of morphine. Lancet 1987, 2, : 723-724.

KRAKOWSKI I, METZ R, BRIQUEL F, GRILLOT M, WATELET M, TRECHOT P. Les opaciacés en cancérologie: aspects récents. Le concours médical 1986, 108 : 1253-1260

MITTERSCHIFFTMALER G, THEINER A, HETZELH, FUITH LC. Analgesic effects of calcitonin in terminal cancer patients. VI Annual Meeting of the European Society of Regional Anaesthesia, Paris, 1985, Abstract Booklet, 76.

PHILIPPS H. Orthopedic surgery. Clinics in Oncology 1984, 3,75-87.

PICHARD E. La codéine en cancérologie. Gaz. Méd., 1987, 94 : 55-57.

TWYCROSS RG. Strong narcotic analgesics. Clinics in Oncology, 1984, 3, 109-133.

VENTAFRIDDA V, RIPAMONTI C, DE CONNO C, BIANCHI M, PAZZUCONI F, PANERAI AE. Antidepressants increase bioavailability of morphine in cancer. Lancet 1987, 1 : 1204.

DIGITAL PRINT
Imprimerie - Photogravure
94851 IVRY / SEINE Tel. : 45 21 03 51

Printed in FRANCE